Victory Is Ahead

Dare to Hope

Facing Childhood Leukemia and the Unexpected

Elisa D. Marchetti

Victory is Ahead
by Elisa Marchetti
© 2022 by Elisa Marchetti
All rights reserved.

Editing: Dr. Yvette Rice, LLVE, LLC
Cover Design by Jan Hammond
Typesetting by Inktobook.com
Published by: Amanda Goodson Global, LLC

Printed in the United States of America
ISBN (Hardcover): 978-1-951501-35-8
ISBN (Paperback): 978-1-951501-33-4
ISBN (eBook): 978-1-951501-34-1

Endorsements

Elisa Marchetti invites you inside a journey with her family that begins with her son's diagnosis with Leukemia. She shares her pain, her hope, her laughter, and her faith. Her writing shares her struggles with the life-changing events that happened during this three-year journey, but it also shares multiple times where the light breaks into the darkness, and she is renewed in her strength and her hope. It is an authentic, faith-inspired, hopeful journey with her son and her husband through the diagnosis of childhood cancer, the long, difficult road of treatment, and into a future beyond cancer.

Pastor Neil E. White
Rejoice Lutheran Church
Frisco, Texas

Elisa's book, *Victory is Ahead*, is an encouragement to anyone who has faced cancer, but particularly to those who have walked the road with a child. Elisa has faced the demon with her child and husband. As a cancer survivor, I never thought of my cancer as a demon or a person, but it is! It takes up residence in every aspect of your life. What an encouragement to know victory is ahead, and Jesus is with us every step of the way. Elisa has captured the essence of the engagement, fight and triumph over the disease and the spiritual battle. I once again have deep joy in my heart and thank God for past, current, and future victories.

Ilene Bezjian, Doctor of Business Administration
Pancreatic Cancer Survivor
Mount Pleasant, North Carolina

Grab your tissues and prepare your heart to be encouraged! *Victory is Ahead*, is a faith-filled, heart-felt invitation to dare to hope during uncertainty, during sorrow, and during pain while always pointing up.

Pastor Austin Kraft
Grace Fellowship Church
Gypsum, Colorado

Note from the Author

The events depicted in this book are related as I remember them. Others may have a different recollection. I did my best not to misrepresent anyone or any event in any way. I chose, in some cases, not to use individuals' full names to not call attention to them in any way they did not wish.

Dedication

To my husband, Alex, and my son, Sal.
You are my brave warriors. I love you both fiercely.

Table of Contents

Foreword

L ooking at the history of childhood cancer, there are many successes to be seen. Collaborative childhood cancer research over the last 7 decades has vastly improved treatment options, and many children with cancer can now be cured. In the 1960s, survival rates for a child with cancer were in the single digits. Now, a majority of children will survive their cancer – but these successes come at a cost. Children endure short-and long-term side effects of intensive and harsh treatments. And despite all of the progress made, there is still much work to do. At this time, there are still some childhood cancers for which there are no known curative therapies. As a pediatric nurse practitioner who has been caring for children with cancer for 25 years, I have witnessed many advances, but I also never forget that we need to keep advancing to help every child.

Any time a child receives a cancer diagnosis, the entire family is plunged into crisis. Parents in these trying circumstances often experience a wide range of emotions, including shock, fear, anger, anxiety, and sadness. There is no right or wrong way for a parent to feel, and emotions can change from day to day (and even moment to moment) over the course of a child's illness and treatment. Parents must find ways to cope with their own emotions and stress, learn about their child's illness and the treatment needed, help their child to adjust and deal with what is happening to them, prepare to care for their child when they are able to go home and communicate about what is happening to their extended family and friends. In short, there are many competing responsibilities and tasks which would be challenging at the best of times, but are completely overpowering during one of the most devastating situations a parent can face. I meet families during one of the most stressful times of their lives. I met the Marchetti family at such a time in the summer of 2018, shortly after their son Sal was diagnosed with leukemia. This book is

Lisa's story of her personal journey through her child's cancer diagnosis and treatment.

A child's cancer diagnosis affects every member of the family and can have significant impact on the family's overall functioning. In the midst of Sal's cancer treatment, the family endured another devastating blow as cancer affected their family for a second time. Lisa details many aspects of her experience with both her child's and her husband's cancers, and shares practical advice built from her experience. In addition, she details how her faith was instrumental to her in navigating the often bumpy course—and the many uncertainties—of their family's journey through two cancer diagnoses.

What started as a journal to help Lisa find solace and strength has developed into this book–a tangible way for Lisa to share her experience and wisdom with other caregivers who are in similar situations. A diagnosis of cancer is overwhelming, and families need resources and avenues of support to help them find their way through. This book is an offering of support to other families in their time of need, from a mother who has been on the front lines of her own family's battle with cancer.

Mrs. M, "Super Sal's" nurse practitioner

Acknowledgments

I am grateful for my husband and son and their support of this book. Alex, your love for me is shown in many ways and I am humbled to be your wife. Thank you for loving me. I continue to lean on your wisdom, strength, and perseverance. Sal, you are resilient and brave. I love being your mom and am so grateful to God for you, and all that you are, and who you will become. You have a gift to see the intangible power and love of God in the world, and I pray that it goes with you for the rest of your life.

To my parents. My mom, Kathy, and deceased father, Pastor Dan. They inspired who I am today through their unshakable faith in Jesus, their love for adventure, and their gift of service. They both were critical during Sal's cancer journey and played an important role. They were the first to remind me of Deuteronomy 31:8, which was our lifeline. My mom continued to sacrificially love and serve our family through her own grief and shared in the role of a caretaker. My mom has a gift where I never had to ask her to help me as she already knew what to do and how to fill the gaps. I love her deeply.

I want to especially thank my sister, Mandy, and her family. She was an anchor for me and never far away. She came to Sal's appointments with us before the pandemic, and nothing was out of reach for me to ask her for. She felt and knew the intricate details of the disappointments and always brought a secure hope to never lose sight of knowing God is still writing Sal's story.

I want to recognize both of my brothers, Steve and Jeff, and their families. Their tremendous support and rallying together as a family was felt by us and gave such encouragement to keep running the race. I especially want to thank my brother Jeff for his help with web design and technology.

Thank you to my in-laws, Ken and Jackie Marchetti, along with my sister-in-law Christie Roberts and her family. You paused your own life when we needed you and visited us multiple times in Texas to offer your support and help. Your prayers were felt across state lines, and we knew you were rooting for us the entire time. Thank you for being prayer warriors.

I want to recognize Dr. Amanda Goodson, my amazing mentor. She was an answer to prayer during a transitional time, and I have no doubt God brought us together for many reasons. She gave me sound guidance and ongoing encouragement. This book would not have been possible without her – she gave me the ultimate gift–her time and wisdom. I can never express how grateful I am for her.

I am thankful for my editor, Dr. Yvette Rice. This final version would not be possible without your expertise and prayerful method. This book has the fingerprints of many people who supported it along the way, and you were a true gift to me. Your partnership was so very appreciated and meaningful. Thank you for your time and investment in this story.

I would like to thank my Pastor, Neil White, and the people of Rejoice Lutheran Church in Frisco, Texas. Pastor Neil and his wife, Carissa, walked with our family during the trials, showing us steadfast commitment and support. They both came to the hospital multiple times and brought joy to Sal and our family. Rejoice Lutheran Church wrapped its arms around us from the moment we heard the news. The quilting ladies made quilts for Sal, and meals were provided. They have continued to support us through a toy drive for children with cancer each year. Our church family was a pillar of support for us, and we are so very grateful.

Lastly, I want to recognize the doctors and nurses at Children's Medical Center hospital in Dallas and Plano, Texas. I can never express how your care, expertise, and compassion made an impact on us. Despite facing Childhood Cancer, the hospital became a special and cheerful place for us because of you. You became our family in the trenches with us. You also never stopped believing and hoping for a cure. We thank you for your incredible quality of care and your impact.

Introduction

The Greatest Deception

I am the greatest deception of all time. More than 400,000 families worldwide experience the ominous, fateful, and brewing storm I bring each year.[1] I know you and your DNA better than you. I can mimic a perfect copy from within your cells, but it's not really you...it's me, the *Great Deceiver*. I am cunning, ruthless, and smart. Seems like I am always one step ahead. But, as with all great triumphs, this will become my greatest downfall from victory.

I go by many names, but you may know me as... *Childhood Cancer.*

The battle is almost here. Can you feel it? Don't say anything. You'll ruin the shock. I need to keep a low profile and go undetected. I know it's only a matter of time before I am discovered…but that's ok because my work has already begun.

Do you see his parents sitting on the couch in the hospital hallway? I am there too, watching and waiting with my foul smile. The white walls are a contradiction to my darkness. My archrival is here too. There it is in the shadows; that relentless, reckless, and stubborn flicker… *the flicker of hope*. I can't seem to overtake it. For the light always shows up. We both know that eventually, I will be overthrown. But of all days, here it is again…*the flicker*.

Look closer at his mom. They all have the same look, complete and utter sorrow. If this goes according to my plan, I will make her doubt everything about herself, including her motherhood. However, the flicker will want to sway her. There is a power she will find and strength in her that she never knew she had. And look, his dad. He is the protector. I can tell he takes his job seriously. His dad has his arm around his wife with care and is looking at her, not the doctor. He will want more than anything to protect his family from this pain…his little boy, his wife, who he vowed to protect. No matter how hard he tries, I've designed it intentionally; he can't protect either of them from this pain and suffering. But, the flicker will sway him too. There is another form of protection and security he will bring to his family.

Their life is about to change forever. If I am successful, I will wreck everything they hold dear. I will ruin their careers. Those are usually the first to go, but that's not even the worst of it. It crumbles quickly after that. Next will be their marriage, their son, their future and ultimately, what I have come to steal is their light,

> **What I have come to steal is their light, their flicker...** *their hope.*

their flicker... *their hope.* It's *go* time. This is my moment! They are about to find out who I am. The doctor is about to speak slowly, and the words will be deafening. I will silence my voice and gradually fade into the background as the chain of events moves forward.

"Alex, Lisa, unfortunately, it is what we expected... Your child has cancer."

The words hit like a punch in the very pit of my core. It's a clean knock-out as I try to gather what is left of the pieces of my heart and somehow rise again to face the enemy within my son... *cancer.*

In 2018, as other families began their summer plans,

ours suddenly took a different turn as our plans disappeared, and our cancer journey began. Our fun-loving and animated son, Sal, was diagnosed with Acute Lymphoblastic Leukemia when he was 6 years old. He had just finished kindergarten with big hopes and dreams of what awaited. My husband, Alex, and I had ideas of what kind of childhood we wanted to give him; however, our lives changed instantly. The doctors told us this would be about a 3-4 year journey on active chemotherapy. That reality was crushing to hear. Sal was facing a life-threatening road ahead, and even in the best-case scenario, he would be about 10 years old when this was finished; and likely seeing doctors for the rest of his life. The childhood hopes and dreams we once held now vanished.

Within 9 months of Sal's diagnosis, more unimaginable news came. My dad unexpectedly died and went to heaven. For those who have lost a parent, you will understand. My dad was my teacher of life, he was the one who shared with me the love of Jesus, and above all, he loved my mom so deeply. Both my parents together were my greatest role models. They lived with us for five months during Sal's early phase of treatment as they redirected their life and moved to Texas from Colorado to help us when we heard those soul-crushing words, "Your child has cancer."

And then, the one-two punch, the soul-crushing words returned. Alex, my husband, was diagnosed with cancer less than a year later. The news was devastating. *Both my son and my husband were facing the same enemy.* Alex, my hard-working husband, the one I looked to when times were hard, the one who loved me since high school, my rock now was facing Pancreatic Cancer. He was 37 years old at the time. It was only caught by the grace of God. Alex is always the one to bring humor through his witty observations or satire. He keeps us laughing with each other through the many trials, and leads our family through his discerning

Both my son and my husband were facing the same enemy.

wisdom...now, he too was facing a storm. My husband's journey was about a year of recovery that took sharp twists and turns around every corner *simultaneously during our son's chemo treatments.* As I am writing this book, both my son and husband have now finished their treatments and are in remission, and I can say Halleluiah! We celebrate their "Victory."

Let me pause for a moment as you might be thinking, *how did you manage through that?* Well, to be honest, it was survival. Day by day, moment by moment. You might be thinking, this title is misleading, Victory? Yeah, Right…What Victory? There were many moments of tears (if a person had a max threshold of the number of tears in a lifetime, I probably would have met it already). There was immense worry, fear, anxiety, and grief. There were also moments of joy that I didn't think were possible and strength that rose from the darkness. During that time, I could not imagine but some of our most incredible family memories were from the hospital room. Relationships were formed that were life-changing and growth in surprising and abundant ways.

I am sharing my experience with you so that you know you are not alone. There is nothing glamorous about cancer. Prayer is our battle strategy. We hold onto God's promises and run the race holding on to our faith in Jesus Christ. We may never know "why"; my heart grieves with those, and all that cancer took. For those who just started a life-threatening journey for your child or are in the middle of it, we are cheering for you. We remain humbled, encouraged, and hopeful for a cure one day!

Introduction: The Greatest Deception

We have a God of peace (during uncertainty)
We have a God of joy (during sorrow)
We have a God of miracles (during pain)

With confidence, we have HOPE and VICTORY ahead.
God is with you through this:

Lisa

Notes

1   "Cancer Statistics," *Childhood Cancer Facts, St Jude Children's Research Hospital*, accessed January 14, 2022, https://www.stjude.org/treatment/pediatric-oncology/childhood-cancer-facts.html#:~:text=Cancer%20Statistics,now%20become%20long%2Dterm%20survivors.

Chapter 1

Trauma: The Unimaginable Comes True

…I am the voice of trauma.

I am numbing to your core, and many times I am often misunderstood and mislabeled. I am branded as stomach aches, headaches, shock, and denial but make no mistake, it's all me. I am trauma. Some say I hideout and then can pounce quickly with no preparation. Others say I am with them constantly. Just wearing them down slowly and even as they try to push me away, I am always there clinging close to the surface, ready to come up. My impact will be felt for years. But don't lose hope; even in the darkest places I have been, I always seek and look for the light. As that is the only way home.

Something is not right. But, what? What could this be?

The Lord our God said to us at Horeb, "You have stayed long enough at this mountain."

Deuteronomy 1:6 NIV

Something is not right with my son. There is anguish in the air. I keep asking myself, "Why didn't the doctor call yet?" My son, Sal, is lying on the couch, lethargic and limp. His small 6-year-old frame is so thin, and I can see his eyes are closed but his body is not resting. His breathing is so heavy, almost like he can't get air, and a constant heaving rhythm is in his chest. An unknown and devious enemy is lurking within his cells. We have no way of knowing. My mind is on replay, "Something is terribly wrong. But, what! What is it?" The unknown is soul-gripping. My laptop is open, just trying to catch up on work emails, but my mind is elsewhere, and thoughts are circling. I hear Alex, my 6'2, strong framed, teddy bear-like husband, quietly walk through the garage door in his hospital scrubs as he just got home from Dallas Children's hospital, where he was working today. He is a medical device rep for multiple hospitals. Dallas Children's Hospital has always been a favorite for him. "That's a nice surprise, I am glad he got home early," I think to myself. "No call yet," I yell down the stairs. I can tell he is concerned by the way he pauses his movements for that split second when I yell down, and he listens intently. Other than my son's breathing, the house is quiet and still. It's pure agony.

"Buzz Buzz," My cell phone rings, and it sends a relief to my core, "Finally," I think to myself, and simultaneously I have a nerve-wracking feeling. Something is very wrong. I say, "hello." The nurse on the other line has no pleasantries, and her tone is alarming and curt. "Is this the parent of Salvatore Marchetti?" "Yes!" I reply quickly. There is no glimmer of hope in her voice. She says in a commanding yet concerned way,

"You cannot wait. You need to go! Do you understand? You need to go now!"

"You need to take him to the ER immediately. The blood test results came back. We have called ahead to the Plano Children's hospital, and they have a room ready for you. You cannot wait. You need to go! Do you understand? You need to go now!"

3

I quickly hang up and hurry to the other room where Alex looks prepared and ready to process whatever words are about to come out. He was an EMT early in our marriage. I can tell he is trained to be calm under pressure, and his movements are slow and controlled. On the other hand, I am moving fast and uncontrolled as my arms and body shift anxiously. I feel so terrified and confused, but somehow I manage to speak, and my words are clear and unshaken, "Something about his blood count. We need to go. They said we need to go right now!" The lump is forming in my throat, and I feel panic swooping in. Nothing makes sense. I send a quick text to my mom and sister, "Just Pray. Heading to the ER." My husband, the constant calm in the storm, carries our son to the car without difficulty. He gives me his look. The look I know so well. His dark brown eyes are both gentle and determined at the same time. They give me stable confidence and are full of trust.

He says calmly, *"C'mon, let's go."*

Life changes in an instant. It was almost as if the words in Deuteronomy were written for us, *"You have stayed long enough at this mountain." …Go! Get moving.* Written by Moses, this verse comes from Deuteronomy, the fifth book in the Bible. It is filled with God's promises, covenant, and commitment to the Israelites. God shares through Moses the great Ten Commandments and ways of living a fulfilling life. He shows them what it means to be called His chosen people. It is loaded was God's promises for us, even in today's age. The scripture is a specific moment of transition for the Israelites. They had already been through other battles and were on the mountain. These are the words of the Lord, "You have stayed long enough on this mountain," and the command to get moving. So, they went, following their leader Moses, with God at the helm facing the next giant ahead without stopping.

Similar to our life, the nurse's words rang in my ear "You cannot wait; you need to go, now!" The trajectory changed; there was no going back. God had set the Israelites apart for such a journey, and He, too, had set us apart. So, we followed the path ahead with God at the helm. Facing the giant of cancer ahead without stopping...*while still holding onto hope.*

When the Unexpected Diagnosis Happens

"The Lord himself goes before you and will be with you; he will never leave you nor forsake you. Do not be afraid; do not be discouraged."

Deuteronomy 31:8 NIV

5

We arrive at Children's Hospital in Plano, Texas. The ER is crowded as my husband carries our son in his arms. We immediately get assigned a room, and every nurse who walks in gives us a look of compassion. They know something we don't know. I can tell by how they provide us with comfort and care in the best way possible. Alex and I are given water and coffee. There is such sympathy in their voices. I will never forget the kind-heartedness shown by complete strangers, even before we knew what was happening.

My older sister, Mandy, shows up in the ER unexpectedly. She knew to come before I even needed to ask. Sisters are like that. She is tall and slender with light brown hair and brown eyes. We look nothing alike on the outside, but our hearts are connected on the inside. She is five years older than me, and growing up, she always looked out for me and protected me. She brings Sal a stuffed animal, and he cracks a smile. She brings Alex a tea, and a smile follows as well. She then takes some more goodies out of her purse and hands me a Diet Coke and a Slim Jim. I can't help but laugh…something I had not done in a while. She knows me so well…my favorite snacks. Even here, in this place, she is looking out for me. We haven't eaten anything, and the nourishment she brings is welcomed and appreciated.

The ER doctor comes, pulls up a chair, and calmly sits directly in front of me. She has my full attention, and she speaks slowly and spells out the path forward. I don't remember a lot of what she said, except *three* things ring in my head:

1. "We need to start a blood transfusion on Sal immediately so he can get oxygen to his heart," *...I think to myself – "Got it, they are very concerned about his heart."*

2. "A nurse paramedic ambulance is on the way as we need to transport you to Dallas Children's Hospital because we don't have the expertise here given the test results." *...I am almost shouting to myself in my head, "Ok, got it, just tell me! What, What are the test results!"*

3. "There are several more tests needed to confirm, but one of the things we are testing is for Leukemia" *....My brain freezes. She keeps talking, and I see her mouth is moving, but I don't hear another word. I am stuck on Leukemia. Time freezes. "Wait, What? That means cancer, right? No, No, No!"*

And then suddenly, time resumes. My ears return, and I'm in the room again, hearing the sounds, the beeping, and the hustling noise. Ok, I'm here, I am following her, and I've caught back up. Her lips move again, and I hear the following words come out. "You should be aware, once you get to Dallas Children's hospital, you will be on the...*oncology floor.*" All sounds stop again, but her lips keep moving. Gosh darn it, she did it again...my brain freezes. I see my sister looking at me with sympathy and sadness in her eyes. Time has stopped, and I am stuck for a second time on the word *oncology*...this means cancer, right? Nothing is making sense.

....My brain freezes. She keeps talking, and I see her mouth is moving, but I don't hear another word. I am stuck on Leukemia. Time freezes.

We load up into the ambulance. I am in the front seat, and Sal is in the back. Only one adult is allowed, so Alex plans to follow behind in the car. Plus, he needs to go back to the house and pick up a few things for me; as they shared, Sal would be hospitalized for several days. It turns out that it is eight days we will initially spend in the hospital. I glance in the back of the ambulance to see Sal. I can't see much, but I can hear some talking and lots of beeping and different sounds. I

8

look out my window and see my sister and my husband standing next to each other with one arm around each other as we drive away. I am living out my greatest fear. I wave to them both trying to prove to myself I am going to be strong; we got this, it's all going to be fine. I'm sure my eyes reveal the truth, "I'm petrified,"...and off we go.

We arrive at Dallas Children's Hospital, and the elevator opens as the EMT and nurse paramedic push my son on the gurney. I follow behind and could see several tubes and an oxygen mask on my son. I feel small and unfamiliar in this big hospital. I follow, trusting in those who know the way to the right floor and our right room. By this time, it's late at night, but a hospital is never quiet or still. I am naturally a shorter person, barely up to 5' 3", but I feel even smaller...almost invisible at that moment. I am living another life as I watch the patient on the gurney. The patient is my one and only son, my child...my Sal. The smell of newly cleaned disinfectant surrounds us. A smell I soon would crave for comfort and a feeling of safety. The first thing that caught my eye was the white walls in big writing that read, "Welcome to the Gill Center of Childhood Cancer and Blood Disorders." Seeing the word Childhood Cancer packs the same punch. Questions, thoughts, and emotions are running through my head at a million miles a minute…

My mind was spinning but in my heart – I was almost numb and couldn't pray.

is this really my life? What am I doing here? What is going to happen? Surely this isn't happening; Sal will be better in a few days. My mind was spinning but in my heart – I was almost numb and couldn't pray. There was no emotion. You have to understand; *prayer is my sustenance.* I grew up in the church as a Pastor's kid and prayer was my lifeline, this is what I knew to do…the very thing that was my life, I could not do.

At that very moment, I was merely a shell. I learned at that moment, why the church and body of believers are God's loving and merciful design not for His needs but for each of us and our needs when our earthly bodies fail us or when our emotional strength is crippled. We were never meant to walk alone – *and we don't have to.* Even though I could not pray, I felt hope and strength from the prayers of others. We had reached out to our Pastor earlier in the day, and our church community, Rejoice

Lutheran Church, became a pillar of support from that moment on. Many people were praying for us, and I felt it, and those prayers mattered. Nothing could have prepared me for what was ahead, although only as God can; God was preparing us and orchestrating what we would need for the next three and half years. *Deuteronomy 31:8 NIV "Do not be afraid; do not be discouraged."*

This verse in Deuteronomy has been a theme throughout our journey *Deuteronomy 31:8 NIV "The Lord himself goes before you and will be with you; he will never leave you nor forsake you. Do not be afraid; do not be discouraged."* A constant reminder that God goes before us and is with us. God views

We were never meant to walk alone – *and we don't have to.*

every situation through the eyes of victory. Although the trajectory pivoted and we were now moving into the throws of battle, He reminds us with tremendous grace that He goes before us to make our way straight and is always with us. At this verse in Deuteronomy, the Israelites were also at *a new pivot point.*

The succession from Moses to the new appointment leader, Joshua, began. Joshua was to lead them into the entrance of the Promised Land and the readiness for multiple battles. They knew the war was imminent, yet they did not know how God would deliver them. Joshua was expected to lead. The pressure must have been enormous. He was chosen by God for this very task, yet the answers were not yet provided to him. I remember wanting to know the answers, yet they were not provided to us either. We needed to faithfully run our race and complete the task set before us. How did Joshua feel at that moment? Was his mind racing? Was he scared, prepared, maybe even numb? I know how I was feeling. Below is an excerpt from my journal after the initial shock.

July 1, 2018 (Journal Entry)

It's been 2 days since we have had the results and confirmed Leukemia. He is my fun-loving, brave, resilient little boy. I have never felt fear like I do now and continue to say that God is with us and goes before us, but at the same time, I find myself having difficulty praying at times like this. God has prepared us for this with the little blessings and orchestrated support along the way that I didn't even know existed.

God has prepared us with family nearby and my parents, who are now retired. He has prepared Sal's heart and given him a spirit of positivity and fun. And, I know he has prepared me too. I am so thankful for our Pastor and church community. When I haven't been able to pray, I know the community of believers and the prayer warriors in places, in many unexpected places, are thinking and praying for us.

People keep saying that Alex and I are strong and "stay strong," but what does that mean? This is just raw hardship, and I don't even know what strong looks like right now. The short-term plans I had for Sal have halted, and life has changed forever. Alex and I are positive, we are hopeful, we are saved by the Blood of Jesus, and we are changed. Perspectives have changed. Going home and picking up a few things yesterday showed me how different I have become in just the past few days. I walked into the same house with the same stuff and memories, but it felt different. I went into Sal's room. His clothes were on the floor, and his bed was unmade with his blankets scattered. The last couple of nights before going to the ER have been hard. I just wanted to preserve this moment, preserve the innocence, and cherish it in my heart. The next time we come home will be with Sal after chemo treatments and constant fear of infection.

My heart reached out in prayers to the one who knows the answers...

"God, Yahweh,...the doctors and nurses do so much, but you ultimately heal. I fall at your feet, weeping. We will walk this journey, but you can't let us down."

"You need to stay holding our hands every step of the way. Don't become silent. Give us greater faith in you and trust. We are leaning on you as our rock and backbone. I cannot do this without your help."

....I felt the confident nudge from Yahweh, *"I will hold your hand; get ready."*

I'll share with you that I have never referred to God as "Yahweh" in my prayers before this moment. It was strange and unusual for me to reference Yahweh as a name for The Lord. It is not a common name we use at our church; although growing up as a Pastor's kid, I had heard it referenced as another name of God, it was still very rarely spoken. Why was that revealed to me through the Holy Spirit? At first, I didn't understand.

Looking back in my journal, I had to further study why I had written Yahweh. Through additional study, I have learned that Yahweh is the name of God from the Old Testament, back in the time of Moses. It was revealed to Moses in Exodus 4. The Hebrew letters are YHWH which does not include vowels and means Lord (or

Adonai). There is a reverence and sacredness in the name YHWH (Yahweh). It means "I am who I am." Yahweh is sovereign. By using the name Yahweh, God was subtly comforting and reminding me, *"I am* the Lord," and He is in control. God meets us where we're at, and although I maybe did not realize it at the moment or was not fully able to comprehend what was happening, God lovingly reveals His promise and sovereignty. A connection to the promise of Deuteronomy 31:8… "I go before you, I will never leave you or forsake. *I am* Yahweh. The great "I am"…*I am* the one who made you; you are my child. *I am* the one who made Sal. He is my child too. *I am* the one who made Alex. And, *I am* the one who has made your family for this time. Get Ready. You've been on this mountain long enough….*I am*…always with you."

Perhaps you are facing a similar journey or know someone who is; please know *Yahweh, Our Lord,* goes before you and is with you. He is sovereign and in control. He *made* you and your child. You are His. You are not alone. If you feel numb, overwhelmed, confused, or simply can't pray…I've been there too, yet we will still dare to have HOPE ahead.

_____

How did we get here? The Path Leading Up to Leukemia

"Therefore put on the full armor of God, so that when the day of evil comes, you may be able to stand your ground, and after you have done everything to stand. Stand firm then, with the belt of truth buckled around your waist, with the breastplate of righteousness in place, and with your feet fitted with the readiness that comes from the gospel of peace. In addition to all this, take up the shield of faith, with which you can extinguish all the flaming arrows of the evil one. Take the helmet of salvation, and the sword of the spirit, which is the word of God."

Ephesians 6:13-17 NIV

About 3,500 children are diagnosed with Leukemia each year in the United States[1]. As critical as the path after Leukemia is, there was the path before diagnosis that had significant milestones along the way. The armor of God was being formed and crafted. We moved from Los Angeles to Texas in 2014 due to a transfer opportunity for my husband's career. Sal was almost 3 years old at the time, and we were excited for a new adventure and a

16

place that felt like home to raise our son. I, too, had career opportunities as well. This was a bit of a leap of faith.

We had no family nearby, our closest family was in Colorado, and we had no friends at first. It was all just new. Within two years, my sister and her family (her husband and three kids) moved to Texas near us, and my parents retired, which gave them more freedom to travel and visit. Sal has always been an energetic child and fun-loving boy. Before chemo, he had blond, almost white hair and greenish/blue eyes, which is a feature he gets from me. Chemo does different things to the body, and one of the side effects was his hair color turning brown – who would have thought? Compared to other kindergartners, he had a thinner and shorter childlike build, but despite his size, he could run fast and make up for it with his big smile & his contagious loud laughter. Sal had an extraverted personality that held a curiosity about life. He is an only child, so seeing cousins and grandparents often was a huge benefit. Little did I realize how much of a support system we would need from all of them as the path ahead began to unfold. These were building blocks of the armor of God coming together.

Fast forward now to the four weeks before the diagnosis, May 2018. Sal was finishing up with kindergarten, and we had many summer plans. He had strep throat twice within a couple of weeks, and his pediatrician changed his antibiotics a few times.

His skin coloring started to look a little pale but then again, nothing too overly concerning as his energy was up, and he was in good spirits with his fun-loving personality. Within about two weeks, he began complaining of leg pain. He said it hurt to walk, which resulted in a trip to the pediatrician, and was shrugged off by our pediatrician as just part of the side effects of having strep throat and could be a pulled muscle. Something was odd, though – I could feel it in my gut but didn't know what it was. The weekend before being diagnosed, he started saying his heart was hurting and he was out of breath. My energetic little boy suddenly couldn't walk, had low-grade fevers, and was very lethargic.

Again, I brought him to the pediatrician's office first thing in the morning but was told there was no appointment until the afternoon. Alex, my husband, and I swapped places, and I went to work, and he stayed home with Sal and took him back to the pediatrician in the afternoon. This is now three visits to the pediatrician's office within one week. I was worried and kept googling what it could be. The pediatrician's office thought we were helicopter parents and hyper-sensitive.

My husband was told to bring him back home and give him Tylenol and if it doesn't get better in a few days, then bring him back in. He felt dismissed by our pediatrician. I felt they weren't listening to us. Have you ever been there? Has anyone out there ever felt this way? Have you ever felt dismissed or ignored by those you depended on for help? Here is how I handled it. In my moment of deep regret and fear, I would cling tightly to the armor of God. God never dismisses our requests. The armor of God can be trusted.

> **God never dismisses our requests. The armor of God can be trusted.**

By Wednesday, he was still not any better, and this time I was ready to go *full version* Mama Bear protective mode. I took him back in and waited for over an hour to see the doctor. Once we saw the doctor, I was adamant that something was not right with my son. He said they would have a blood test done and call us with the results. Three hours later, I got a phone call from the nurse in our pediatrician's office that we needed to go to the ER immediately. Sal's red blood count was 3.5 hemoglobin as cancer had multiplied so quickly it pushed out all the healthy cells. For reference, most adults average around 12-17.5 for their red blood count.[2] These are the cells that carry oxygen to your heart – no wonder he had no oxygen and felt like he couldn't breathe. His heart literally was running out of oxygen. The dots are starting to connect.

In the Plano ER, they did several additional tests and multiple blood transfusions. After we took the ambulance to Dallas Children's hospital, a biopsy was done the next day, and it was confirmed, Leukemia. He would be starting chemo immediately. I got angry and the guilt set in. Why didn't I bring him in sooner? What if the doctor had taken us seriously? Why didn't I push more? Why didn't I trust my gut? If only I had known. I have come to find out that other families have also had this experience. It often goes misdiagnosed or delayed diagnosis.[3] I have had to wrestle with these feelings throughout the journey. I have had to remind myself many times to cling to the Lord. He has fitted us with His armor. He protected Sal even when those we rely on as medical experts made a mistake – they are only human too, and I know there was no ill intent. The Lord was with us, and He is with you too.

We will hold onto the belt of truth and the breastplate of righteousness. Our feet are fitted with the gospel, and we hold onto the shield of faith to extinguish the flaming arrows of cancer. God promises us the helmet of salvation, and we have the sword of the spirit that will offensively move ahead.

If you or someone you know is newly diagnosed, truly recognize that the path leading up to diagnosis can be important data. If you had a delay, you might be trying to forgive yourself or a doctor for not seeing the signs more clearly. Then know, you are not alone. I, too, have wrestled with anger, guilt, and forgiveness. I encourage you to cling to the armor of God for your security.

Allowing Yourself and Others to Process

"I am worn out from groaning; all night long,
I flood my bed with weeping and drench my couch with tears."

Psalm 6:6 NIV

The entire family is shaken when a child is diagnosed with cancer. Every other care in the world fades, and life becomes focused on the child with cancer. Individual identities sometimes go into the background, life revolves around constant cleaning, and there is a

21

continuous state of fear of germs. Each family member carries a weight and has a role to play that no one willingly chooses. The siblings of the child with cancer play significant roles, and it can be very confusing with a complexity of emotions, depending on the age of the siblings. From the moment of diagnosis, time stops, and the world goes on pause because it reminds us of our mortality. It reminds us of a parent's worst fear, your child's mortality. The Psalmist shows the human heart at its moment of hurt and unbearable pain. Grief can hit your very soul, and it is both an emotional pain and a physical pain that you feel in your body. The response to this can be a variety of complex emotions. Reviewing the grief chart, the diagram on the right in the red lines captures what my experience was going through grief. It's all over the place. Yep, that sounds about right. How about for you?

The "stages" originated from Dr. Ross' observations of the experiences of terminally ill patients. It is never a predictable linear line, but grief is multiple emotions simultaneously, and it is very normal to bounce back and forth in the stages.[4]

Stages of Grief

The roadmap you expected: The road you got:

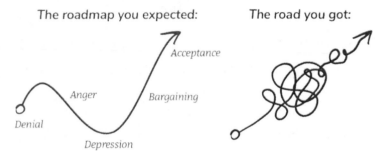

https://speakinggrief.org/get-better-at-grief/

understanding-grief/no-step-by-step-process

I remember lying on the couch, which converts into a couch bed at the hospital. (Side note–One perk about being short is you can sleep in any small space. The hospital couch beds are all tiny…thank you, Lord, for the little things, like making me short!) I remember looking up in the middle of the night with the sounds and machines beeping and tears just flowing uncontrollably. I could not stop. It was a flood of emotion pouring out of my soul. However, not everyone has the same reaction, which is also ok. Perhaps you want to cry, but you just can't. It's still too unbelievable. That's ok too. Below is a poem I wrote for those impacted by Childhood Cancer.

23

To those impacted by Childhood Cancer

To the Moms...

To the moms who knew something was wrong and had to fight for the answers. To the moms, who didn't know what was wrong and felt shocked.

To the moms who are scared and worried but have no choice but to be confident and fearless. To the moms who are confident but still can't sleep.

To the moms who fall on their knees to weep and pray. To the moms who feel overwhelmed and can't pray.

To the moms who kissed that same bald baby head 100 times a day and now kiss their child's bald beautiful head to bring comfort.

To the moms who feel out of control and that life is unkind and ungrateful. To the moms who finally feel she has a sense of purpose and continues to show graciousness and gratitude.

To the moms who relentlessly show up at every appointment and never lose HOPE. To the moms who show up even though they can't stand to see their child suffer and just want this to be over.

To the moms on the Oncology floor. This one is for you. We love you; you are not alone.

To the Dads...

To the dads who drove us to the ER. To the dads who drove to the hospital alone because only one parent was allowed in the ambulance, and he knew I couldn't have my heart broken anymore.

To the dads who were silent, yet their presence brought comfort. To the dads who asked the right questions when we were all speechless.

To the dads who showed strength and calmness, even if inside they weren't. To the dads who felt unprepared and didn't know what to do but demonstrated such tenderness.

To the dads who were emotional when the word "Childhood Leukemia" was confirmed. To the dads who just held their wives, felt numb and couldn't shed a tear.

To the dads who shaved their heads to show solidarity. To the dads who showed it other ways.

To the dads who continue to work and provide when the whole world has gone on pause. They are constantly going to and from the hospital. Their stability, service, and faithfulness to the Lord does not go unnoticed.

To the dads on the Oncology floor. This one is for you. We love you; you are not alone.

To the Nurses...

To the nurses who have seen it all before. To the nurses who see just this one precious child.

To the nurses who give a sense of assurance with a look to a very unsure family. To the nurse who gives a gentle hug or small touch, which demonstrates peace for just a moment.

To the nurse who has to clean it up, again and again, but continues because the patient is stubborn and you know that they are not trying to be difficult, they are really just scared.

To the nurses who see the family's discord and tension and says a prayer for that child. To the nurse who sees a unified family that is strong and will easily overcome.

To the nurse who brings an extra toy just because she knows it will bring a smile. To the nurse who laughs at the patient's joke, which is not funny but, for a split second, helped the pain go away.

To the nurse who is so quiet at night, she is almost like an angel. To the nurse who is loud and boisterous during the day and distracts us from the worry of the world.

To the nurses on the Oncology floor. This one is for you. We love you; you are not alone.

To the Grandmas...

To the grandmas who knew it the second the phone rang. To the grandmas who were not around to answer the phone.

To the grandmas who were able to come and be part of everything. To the grandmas who couldn't physically be there but so desperately wanted to.

To the grandmas that worry for two people; their grandchild and their own child. Their heartstrings tug in every direction.

To the grandmas who do extra cleaning and meals for support. To the grandmas who make quilts and sacrifice in many other ways.

To the grandmas who rush in and may overstep out of love. To the grandmas who are scared to push too hard and add too much pressure, so they love from a distance.

To the grandmas who have just the right words to say and the right time. To the grandmas who are unsure when to speak up and remain quiet yet contain much Godly wisdom.

To the grandmas on the Oncology floor. This one is for you. We love you; you are not alone.

To the Aunts...

To the Aunts who were there every step of the way. To the Aunts that live far away and pray every day for that child.

To the Aunts who google everything about Leukemia and can't stop. To the Aunts that don't want to know the worst because they can't believe this is happening.

To the Aunts who have to tell their own children about their cousin's cancer and don't know what words to use. To the Aunts who have no children, and this niece/nephew will be it for them.

To the Aunts who are a shoulder to cry on when it all feels too much or a phone call away when there is no one else who will understand.

To the Aunts who take you out for a pedicure because you need a break. To the Aunts that bring you coffee in the hospital because you need a mental break.

28

To the Aunts that change plans and take work off to be at appointments and help around the house. To the Aunts that can't, but still give encouragement and support the best they can.

To the Aunts on the Oncology floor. This one is for you. We love you; you are not alone.

To all those impacted when a child has Leukemia. Family, friends, church, neighbors, teachers, community...Don't lose HOPE. This one is for you. We love you; you are not alone.

Shock and grief can be untamed. Give yourself grace and patience, and extend that grace to others on their very first reactions. God is with you, and you are not alone.

Practical Tip – when newly diagnosed

Once you have the diagnosis, identify someone you trust to be the central point of communication. It is physically and emotionally exhausting to be the sole communicator during times of crisis. Below is an easy text or email you can use for those in your inner and outer circle.

"Hi, as many of you now know, our child has been diagnosed with cancer. The first 30-60 days are intense as we start the treatment plan and path forward. I have asked (my sister, mom, friend, etc.) to keep you all updated on our progress. We welcome your prayers at this time and invite you along with us. (My mom, sister, friend, etc.) will be in touch with the needs of our family, as well as updates on our child. I welcome your texts and emails; please understand if I don't respond right away. Thank you!"

Tips and Quotes from Others:

"We started a care bridge site for our daughter. This was the easiest way to keep others informed." (Mom of a daughter who had cancer)

"The 2nd time my daughter was diagnosed we started a personal Facebook page just for my daughter's journey. This allowed us to accept those who we wanted and I posted pictures and was able to document her journey. Looking back it was nice to have a centralized place that showed how far we have come!" (Mom of a daughter who had cancer)

"We rallied the neighborhood kids and put together posters and cards to show our support. This was our way of trying to help as a community as none of us were allowed to go to the hospital" (Neighbor of a child who had cancer)

"The best thing for us is we had a dear friend start a GoFundMe for us as well as provide UberEats Gift cards. This gave us the most flexibly with hospital bills and food choices." (Mom of a daughter who had cancer)

"Cancer is a word no one ever wants to hear. It is especially hard when it's a member of your family, but it was unthinkable that it could happen to my 6-year-old grandson. What could I do to help? I have come to remind myself of three things: First, this is about them, not me. I remember to put my feelings and emotions in check so they could allow their emotions to flow. Secondly, what were ways I could care for them? I can sit at the hospital, make food, clean the house, and show them I love them with big hugs. Thirdly, Pray, Pray, Pray! We've all just entered unfamiliar territory and ask Jesus to lead the way. God brings victory even in cancer." (My mom, Grandma of 6-year-old who defeated cancer)

Notes

1   "Childhood Leukemia," The University of Texas MD Anderson Cancer Center, accessed on September 25, 2021, https://www.mdanderson.org/cancer-types/childhood-leukemia.html.

2   "Hemoglobin Test," Mayo Clinic, Updated October 9, 2019, https://www.mayoclinic.org/tests-procedures/hemoglobin-test/about/pac-20385075.

3   "Diagnosing Childhood Cancer," American Childhood Cancer Organization, accessed on September 11, 2021, https://www.acco.org/diagnosis/.

4   "There is No Step by Step Process," Pennsylvania State Institute, Understanding Grief, accessed on January 11, 2022, https://speakinggrief.org/get-better-at-grief/understanding-grief/no-step-by-step-process.

Chapter 2

Treatment Plan: Day 1 of Healing

…I am the voice of pain.

I am not your enemy, although when you see me, you hate me. I don't blame you for feeling the way you do. Please know that I am just another form of protection that tells you something is wrong. I take on various forms such as throbbing, aching, sharp, and even can pierce your very soul. However, I will not last forever. The suffering I cause is just for a little while. The light is peaking through and is for eternity. There is no victory without me. I know your pain is great right now, but the victory will be even greater!

arning to Trust through the Worry

"Therefore do not worry about tomorrow, for tomorrow will worry about itself. Each day has enough trouble of its own."

Matthew 6:34 NIV

The journey began, and the plan was set in motion. The biopsy was confirmed on Friday, June 29, 2018, and on Monday, July 2nd, within 72 hours of being diagnosed, Sal's port was surgically placed, and he received his first chemo treatment. It was Day 1 of healing. The port used is a standard method to get chemo into the body. It allows drugs to be put directly into the bloodstream quickly and spread throughout the body. Ports eliminate the difficulty of finding veins and help reduce stress and discomfort for the child.[1] There are other ways of administering chemo; however, the port was the best option given the number of infusions Sal would need to have. It is all under his skin, except there are three tiny dots you can see and feel above his upper torso above his chest, and it sticks out slightly. His port was a tangible reminder of hope! Treatment was possible, and how grateful I am for the port. We had a path towards healing.

It was go time! Adrenaline was pumping, and we were running our race and ready to go all in. The general outline of the phases of Leukemia treatment was shared with us, but no details were provided because it all depended on certain milestones that could change the course of his treatment. The first phase is called *"Induction."* The goal of Induction is to aggressively treat cancer and put it in remission within the first 30 days. Multiple different chemotherapies are used, and treatments generally are given through both a port and into the CFS fluid in the spine called a Lumbar Puncture. This first month is intense and requires prolonged hospital stays for treatment and frequent visits to the doctor.[2] This was essentially the first month of treatment. Parents and caregivers are given a new nomenclature, and you begin to speak in acronyms as the foreign language suddenly becomes clear. You now know more than you ever thought you would know about blood cells and how to read medical scans, results, and tests. White blood cells, red blood cells, and platelets all have a significant job in the body. As you learn about these critical components in our blood, you learn how Leukemia starts with a mutation of the white blood cell and then multiplies quickly to push out all the other healthy cells. Chemo is designed to go in and destroy any quick replicating cell. To kill Leukemia, many healthy cells will have to be destroyed along with it. It's a difficult concept to reconcile in a mama's heart.

We were released from the hospital to head home within eight days, which quickly turned into a return trip due to a fever. There is a constant state of "fever watch" when a family has a child with cancer. The orders were that whenever Sal spiked a fever of 100.4 or higher, we called the doctor and would be asked to come into the hospital (or ER if after hours) as the fever was an indication of infection. The hospital protocol is to give antibiotics through the port immediately to get ahead of a potential bacterial infection. Given the compromised immune system, a simple fever could turn critical and extremely serious without antibiotics. We got to the hospital on this particular fever ER visit, labs were drawn, cultures were growing, and it was confirmed that Sal had

> **To kill Leukemia, many healthy cells will have to be destroyed along with it. It's a difficult concept to reconcile in a mama's heart.**

a bacterial infection We knew he would remain in the hospital until the end of Induction (about another three weeks). During this discovery of this infection, it was later deemed he had pseudomonas. The doctors did not know where the source of the infection was, and it was an extremely dire time. They were concerned it would spread, and he would end up in the Pediatric ICU. He was very sick and in pain. We had several doctors and experts assisting us with the path forward and reviewing the multiple obstacles that *could* occur.

One particular day, I recall a severe vibe in the room as they explained to me the options available. One source of the bacteria could be in the port itself, which would require another surgery to remove the port. At this point, surgically replacing the port with a different one would not be a solution as his body would be too weak to heal due to the chemo. So Sal would have a PICC (Peripherally Inserted Central Catheter) line for his chemo instead. This would likely be more extended hospital stays and additional risks of more infections. Another concern was that the infection was in his digestive tract, which could also be very serious.

In addition to chemo, Sal was also on heavy steroids that caused constant hunger. On steroids, Sal would sometimes require two to three snacks in the middle of the night, and the hunger would be overwhelming. The steroids gave him intense cravings, and given all that he was going through, we catered to it. Food was his only joy. He got to order lunch from the TV in the hospital, and they would bring it up to the room. Because he was on steroids, he was allowed double meals and even that was not enough to curve the hunger. Chicken nuggets quickly became his favorite meal. No judgment here, I don't want to admit it, but we even allowed him to order Chicken Nuggets with ketchup for breakfast. If he wanted chicken nuggets for breakfast, in the grand scheme of things, fine with me if this will give him a glimpse of comfort. For those of you with children on steroids right now; let me give you some hope, I promise you, it won't last forever. Just do what you can to survive those intense steroid weeks.

As the plan was beginning to develop, we had a team of several doctors come into the room to share with us a look ahead, and let me tell you, it was not a pretty picture of what we were facing. We had an infectious disease doctor and their intern in the room, the surgeon who may have to remove the port, the oncologist, a nurse practitioner, and medical students. All standing around in a half-circle, with reserved looks on their faces. It was somber. This was not part of the plan, but we now had to adjust. I could see the worry on their faces as they spoke very slowly and had their heads tilted downward. I'm sure my face was dripping with concern and fret with my eyebrows V-shaped and eyes filled with questions...but not the kind of questions they would have the answers to. I could almost feel their apprehension and uneasiness as they all moved in the room and shared the possible "what if" scenarios with me from their lens of expertise. There were no smiles as the candid and harsh reality set in.

Finally, after going through the options and the risks, they asked if I had any questions. I shook my head. They started to scuttle out of the room, and one doctor looked at Sal and asked if he had any questions. He said, "Actually, I do." Suddenly the interns took out their note pads and had their pens ready to write. The team became very alert. There was a flicker of hope that sparked. And Sal said, "So, I've been listening to everything, but I am just wondering if next time, with my chicken nuggets, do you think I can get a little bit more ketchup, please?" Smiles and laughs broke out. He wasn't worried a bit. He just was ready for lunch. The following morning as we were waiting for either good news or bad news on his blood work, one of the interns came up with a cup full of ketchup packs. She said, "We all agreed this might be the best option for him right now." A gentle gift of empathy, care, and laughter during the unknown. I will never forget the thoughtfulness of that jester.

We went through several weeks of additional antibiotics and testing, and thankfully we did not need to get the port removed, and miraculously the infection healed. The worry was for nothing. A small reminder for us that when you are in the depths of fear and facing a road that seems to have no viable solutions, the flicker of hope will not be snuffed out. Maybe, *just maybe*, treat yourself to your version of nuggets and ketchup. For you, it might be an exceptional coffee or an ice cream. It's ok to give yourself permission to have joy even in the most devastating circumstances. The Lord says, *"do not worry about tomorrow; today has enough worries of its own."*

And maybe, just maybe…it's ok to even splurge a little on ketchup.

Hospital Community

The Subculture we didn't choose yet is the community for whom I am forever grateful

"Carry each other's burdens, and in this way you will fulfill the law of Christ."

Galatians 6:2 NIV

The team of doctors and nurses walked side by side with us on this journey and had a crucial role. I remember their kindness, empathy, and compassion. We were thrown into the thrust of a new subculture that I never would have chosen, yet here were the nurses, hospital staff, and even the other families you see in the hallways. You know each other's burdens, and in a small way, it is a place to wrap our virtual arms around each other as we all witness the pain and suffering of our own child.

I remember a couple of experiences that brought me a different perspective and reflections of this new community that was carrying our burdens and gave opportunities for us to carry their burdens as well.

The Playroom

I'll paint the scene for you to imagine. The hospital

playroom on the 6th floor is designed for those on the cancer floor only. Due to fear of infection, it's dedicated to those with cancer or blood disorders. Given the cleaning schedule to reduce the risk of germs, there were only specific times a day when the children could go into the playroom. These were treasured moments in the hospital and were one of the highlights of our day. The playroom had two main sections. One area had small tables and chairs with lots of different crafts, toys, puzzles, games, and pearler beads (which became a favorite pastime). The other area had the coveted air hockey, a TV, and Sal's favorite, video games.

Each child comes in with their parent or caretaker, and each child is connected to tubing connected to a pole with machines on top that are usually two large rectangles about 10-12 inches. The poles have wheels, so you literally wheel this pole around next to your child. Sal, even at times, liked to stand on the legs of the pole and be wheeled around. Oh, the small joys in the hospital. It takes a bit of maneuvering as the pole follows the child and of course…there is beeping from these machines. These machines are wonderful inventions; however, at the same time, there is usually a constant beep for a variety of reasons. It could be there are air bubbles, the tube gets kinked, medication is low, or I believe that these machines have their own personalities and just get grumpy and beep. We had several machines that I felt were just cranky all the time. They are quite finicky devices, so many times, it's simply a false alarm that can get fixed in a matter of seconds. There is probably at least one if not more machines beeping at any given moment, and parents quickly learn how to hit the "ignore" button until a nurse comes to troubleshoot the machine. The "ignore" button is instant relief but only lasts a few minutes, so you are gearing up for another inevitable annoying beeping sound unless the nurse comes immediately. Parents, it's a bit comical. So picture yourself in this familiar scene. Sal and I are in the playroom doing air hockey, and sure enough, someone's machine starts beeping. You quickly scan to see if it's your child. If it's not your child, you give the parent whose child it is a nonverbal smile or a nod, simply saying, "I know how you're feeling...don't worry; next time, it will be us." There is a nonverbal mutual bond and yet a deep understanding as we all relate and, in a true sense, carry each other's burdens – even if that burden is an annoying ill-tempered beeping machine.

Other Cancer Families

Here's another reminder of human connection and carrying each other's burden. It occurred during Sal's initial phase in ALL (Acute Lymphoblastic Leukemia) called Induction. As shared in the previous chapter, we spent most of the Induction phase hospitalized, about four weeks.

During one of the weeks, Sal met a friend, a 5-year-old boy. He had a malignant brain tumor and was further along in this process than Sal needing both chemo and radiation. As the boys played Xbox together in the play-room, naturally, I struck up a conversation with the child's dad. He explained to me that he and his wife have four kids. His wife is home with their infant child while he stays in the hospital with their child with cancer.

Additionally, their oldest has Down's syndrome. This is also called Trisomy 21 and is when a person has an extra chromosome.[3] *Wow, I thought.* Perspective: Just when we start feeling that we are the only ones with cancer, God gently reminds us that others are facing cancer and balancing many family needs. The boys played all week together. Sal's friend was discharged a few days later and got to go home. Although we still had a couple more weeks of hospitalization, this encouraged me that this burden is not ours alone to carry. We don't walk this path alone.

The Girl in the Unicorn Room

Lastly, as I reflect on carrying each other's burdens, another story stands out to me that was early in Sal's treatment, as we were spending weeks in the hospital's four walls and my intimate interaction with a fellow mom.

We do not speak the same language, but we understand each other clearly. The mom speaks Spanish, and I speak English. She is the mom of the girl in the room with the unicorn on her window. Each room in the hospital is decorated with a cartoon or colorful picture on the window. We have spider-man on our window, and it makes us smile, heading to our room…a tangible reminder that we have superheroes around us. Our room is about six doors further down the hallway. Whenever I go to the kitchen area or go to the playroom, we pass the unicorn room. Sal befriended the 10-year-old daughter from the unicorn room in the playroom. She was much further along than Sal and had other complications very noticeable by her physical appearance. We saw her younger sister, who was about 6 years old, often throughout our stay. The mother always had the same look, deep sadness and despair. Her shoulders always seemed hunched over and defeated. She almost seemed withdrawn from her children, and in her eyes, I could tell she was living through the worst-case scenarios of cancer. She almost had hopelessness about her. Her life was what we all were trying to avoid.

I walk into the kitchen area, and the mom of the unicorn room is standing by the microwave. I look at her, and she looks at me. Our eyes meet, and we know each other's torment; no words are needed. I open my arms, and we hug and hold each other as moms for a few minutes. We know each other's pain, worries, and sorrow. This just isn't right; it makes me want to scream! No child should have to go through cancer, let alone my child. It is the most unnatural thing in the world to watch your child suffer. She points to her stomach and refers in Spanish to perhaps the liver or pancreas, which are all ominous signs that the medication or the cancer is now attacking the organs and can be catastrophic. We hug once again and cry on each other's shoulders. There is no judgment. *A complete stranger, but a bond is formed,* and a mutual understanding that no one else gets unless they are going through this battle.

Communication is not always verbal. I didn't have to say one word. I point up to God, and she nods in complete agreement. God is here and is present in this tender moment between two moms.

The next day the 10-year-old girl in the unicorn room was no longer there. I asked a nurse, and she respectfully said, "oh...Umm, she had to go to another place, the hospital, and is very, very sick." I'm not sure what that means, but I know it is not good. I pray for that mom, and if her daughter does not survive, she will rejoice with the Lord Jesus in heaven, and one day, they will be reunited where there is no pain.

God is here and is present in this tender moment between two moms.

The Lord has surrounded us with unique families that have entered our inner circle and will forever be imprinted on our lives in this journey. As you go through this journey or you know someone who is...allow others to carry your burdens when they are too heavy for you. Also, remember that you are there to carry those burdens of others who might need a bit of a lift of hope, encouragement, and a reminder that they are not alone.

Side Effects: Just because the hair grows back doesn't mean it is all better

Whoever dwells in the shelter of the Most High will rest in the shadow of the Almighty. I will say of the Lord, "He is my refuge and my fortress, my God, in whom I trust."

Surely he will save you from the fowler's snare and from the deadly pestilence. He will cover you with his feathers, and under his wings you will find refuge; his faithfulness will be your shield and rampart. You will not fear the terror of night, nor the arrow that flies by day.

Psalm 91:1-5 NIV

Chemotherapy is just what the name sounds likes...it is literally Chemical Medication. It's designed to kill, destroy, and wipe out. The intent is to kill the cancer cells, but collateral damage is in its path; the healthy cells are also affected. Chemo does not know the difference between cancer cells compared to any other fast replicating cells, and so it goes after both healthy and cancer cells. It is a hard thing to reconcile as a parent. Every other time in Sal's life when he felt sick, I would give him medication to make him feel better. If you are a parent, think through the times you gave your child medication. Was it to make them feel better or worse? For us, it would typically be something like cough syrup, Tylenol, or antibiotics. Before cancer, I would even hear myself say, "Take some of this; you will feel better soon." With chemo, it is the complete opposite. You know full well that the medication he will take...*chemo* will make him feel worse. A whole lot worse. You are informed of the short-term side effects and some potential chronic side effects that will impact him for the rest of his life. I would just cling to Psalm 91 during some of the more challenging side-effect weeks. Our refuge is not in the medication...our refuge dwells in the shelter of the Most High, and in Him, we will find rest.

Early in the treatment plan, our doctors share with us the variety of different chemo drugs Sal would be on throughout treatment, and each chemo has its set of side effects. Then to counteract those side effects, you give other medication, which has its own set of side effects. You are in this vicious cycle of trying to balance nausea, pain, digestive impacts, and other random side effects like foot drop, jaw pain, mouth sores, and, of course… we all expect *hair loss*. There is a quote from one of the Facebook Leukemia groups "Just because the hair grows back doesn't mean they are better."

Sal also lost his hair. We knew it, and we expected it. I remember talking with Sal about it as I can imagine it's difficult for anyone to experience their hair falling out, even six-year-old boys. There were clumps, and it started to thin and then he told me, "Mom, I'm ready. Can you shave my head?" It was late at night, and I remember getting the hair clippers out and shaving his precious head, and then, in solidarity, my husband too asked me to shave his head. My brave bald men were very handsome, and I could not be prouder of them both.

> **"Just because the hair grows back doesn't mean they are better."**

It was so visible. Everywhere we went, it was known… my child has *cancer*. I remember walking in the hospital, and it dawned on me how public the hair loss side effect is, yet in the grand scheme of all the side effects, it is the most minor. I would take hair loss any day over some of the other internal side effects. I have been drawn to Psalm 91 as the steady reminder that God is our refuge in times of trouble. He will cover us with His feathers, and under His wings, we are safe. The imagery is beautiful. It's a mother bird protecting its young. Regardless of hair color, texture, or even having no hair at all...God can be trusted. He is our refuge.

When the Plan Changes: Living with Disappointments

"Surely the righteous will never be shaken; they will be remembered forever. They will have no fear of bad news; and their hearts are steadfast, trusting in the Lord."

Psalm 112: 6-7 NIV

There have been many lessons speckled throughout this journey, but I often think about one of the many lessons that we endured: being able to adapt when the plan changes. Living with the disappointments and showing and teaching Sal how to maneuver through life's disappointments was crucial. I remember one specific Thanksgiving. Sal was managing reasonably well, and we were in a phase called Maintenance during his treatment.

51

Maintenance is the fifth phase for Sal and comes after Delayed Intensification, which is one of the most intense phases. This phase aims to destroy any Leukemia cells left in the bone marrow and is about two to three years long.[4] Sal was still immune-compromised; however, the intensity of chemo is lighter in the Maintenance phase than the previous stages. The chemo is still fighting Leukemia but gives the body a chance to recover and "maintain."

We planned to get together with my sister, her family, and my mom. We were hosting! It was going to be a Happy Thanksgiving! ...or so I thought. We had been quarantined the year before, so this was a long-awaited family gathering. This was also the first Thanksgiving since my dad's death, and we wanted to be together. I was so very much looking forward to this time with everyone. Maybe it would be a glimpse of normalcy...a glimpse of having a normal holiday.

Leading up to Thanksgiving, we had a family rule that no one could be sick, even with a cold, for at least two weeks. It was now the Tuesday before Thanksgiving, and no one had been sick – plans were on! It was a go, green light ahead. As most people do, Thanksgiving becomes a family meal of people pitching in for different parts of the meal. My sister's husband proudly does the turkey with a turkey fryer, so they were going to bring the bird, and we planned on doing the ham. The sides were split fairly evenly. She had the dessert; I think I had mashed potatoes. They had stuffing, and we had cranberries and so on. Each of the traditional parts of the meal was covered. It was going to be a feast!

Wednesday at 4 am, the day before Thanksgiving, Sal woke up and had difficulty breathing. It was scary because he spiked a fever. We called the oncologist and went into the hospital. He had croup. Plans immediately changed...Thanksgiving will be alone this year; again... so much for a Happy Thanksgiving. One of our favorite nurse practitioners asked Sal if he was feeling crappy, so with his humor and a smile, he wished her and us a "Crappy Thanksgiving," it was indeed fitting that year. A new nickname for Thanksgiving was given.

When we got home, I quickly realized we had ingredients for half a meal, and my sister had the other half. I called her and shared the news. The feeling of disappointment is different from other feelings because it captures such a letdown and has an element of loss of control. If you are sad, you can think of something to cheer you up. If you are angry, then think through what is triggering the reaction. The thing with disappointment is you don't have control to change the outcome. There is no "go back" or "redo." It's simply dealing with life when the plans change – it is out of our hands. Have you ever had to deliver disappointing news? You know that it will be hard to share and you, too, are disappointed just saying it? Or maybe, you were the receiver of crushing disappointing news. How did you react? Think of the last time you experienced a gut-wrenching disappointing situation. It gets me in the pit of my belly, and there is no hiding it on my face. Here is how I managed through it. The Psalmist acknowledges that bad news is part of life and redirects us to our true north – our hearts are steadfast, trusting in the Lord. This verse resonates with me because I have struggled with the fear of bad news. Every appointment, every twist and turn along the way…I didn't want the plan to change – I wanted to only hear the *happy news*. Just tell me the good stuff but leave out the bad stuff. I wanted clarity and control

> **The thing with disappointment is you don't have control to change the outcome.**

of this journey, and only if we could skip to the happy parts. God reminds us to trust Him even in the "bad news."

My sister knew the disappointment the minute I called her. She shared the news with her family, and that Thanksgiving became known as…*Crappy Thanksgiving.* I think Sal got a huge kick out of wishing people a "Crappy Thanksgiving" with a big smile on his face. We managed through the holidays and learned yet again how to deal with disappointments that come our way. It's ok to feel disappointment and even recognize it with a new nickname.

> **God reminds us to trust Him even in the "bad news."**

As the Psalmist reminds us, we will continue to trust and not fear bad news. I really do wish you and your families a Happy Thanksgiving this year, but if you are living a year of Crappy Thanksgivings…I get it; I've been there. If you had wonderful plans in place and now, unfortunately, have ended up with only half of a Thanksgiving dinner, that might not even count as a real Thanksgiving. I get it; I've been there. If you got the news that your child has croup and anxiety is just peeking around the corner… I get it; I've been there. I hold onto Psalm 112 and cling to God's word. We will not be shaken. We are trusting in the Lord because we know there is Victory ahead.

Practical Tip–during Treatment

Being organized can be a challenge. There are so many different medications, hospital bills, and calendar appointments that can easily get confusing. We had a few tools that helped our family.

1. First, my mother-in-law bought a small portable file organizer for us. I organized all the different paperwork – which was a huge help.

2. Secondly, we also had a large family calendar posted visibly for everyone in the household to see that marked the chemo dates and pills. We had stickers that Sal could put on important days, enabling him to be part of the planning. This allowed for greater alignment in communication and awareness. I think the calendar was one of the most helpful tools for Sal as he was at the age where he could follow along, and it helped reduce the anticipation and nervousness.

3. And lastly, we had an app on our phones to help track when Sal needed to take his medication, so we didn't forget or assume the other parent gave him the pills. This allowed our communication to be aligned as caregivers. The one we used was Medisafe; however, there are more out there that you can also demo to see if it works for you. Let the technology help you.

Tips and Quotes from Others:

"I recommend saving all your medical bills, food receipts, parking, and mileage as this can be tax-deductible at the end of the year depending on how you file your taxes." (Tax advisor who specializes in unique tax situations)

"My husband and I share an app "The Cozi Family Calendar" which allowed us to update any changes to doctor appointments and balance the activities of our other children." (Mom of a son with cancer)

"It was completely overwhelming at first. I couldn't keep it all straight, so we dedicated a corner of the counter just for his pills and medications and got a weekly pillbox that allowed for us to separate his medications into specific times a day. This helped but it was still hard to manage." (Mom of a son with cancer)

"One of my ways of showing support is that I tried to keep up with what was going on in treatment so they didn't need to keep repeating it. Sometimes the treatment can move really quickly so when a new word or terminology was shared, I would jot it down and look it up later so I can keep up. I also tried to listen intently so I knew the key names of doctors or nurses as these became trusted relationships. I knew I couldn't always be there but committed to keeping up as a way of showing my support." (My sister)

So, to wrap up, allow yourself to find the right organizing and support system for you as these are just a few that worked for us and others. I encourage you to be thoughtful with your own organizational system as it will help be a stress reliever during treatment.

Notes

1   Nancy Keene, *Childhood Leukemia: A Guide for Families, Friends, and Caregivers (5th Edition)* (Washington: Childhood Cancer Guides, 2018), 153.

2   "Treating Children with Acute Lymphoblastic Leukemia," *American Cancer Society*, accessed on September 11, 2021, https://www.cancer.org/cancer/leukemia-in-children/treating/children-with-all.

3   "Facts about Down Syndrome," *Center for Disease Control and Prevention (CDC)*, updated on April 6, 2021, https://www.cdc.gov/ncbddd/birthdefects/downsyndrome.html.

4   "Acute Lymphoblastic Leukemia Chemotherapy Phases," *About Kids Health*, updated on March 6, 2018, https://www.aboutkidshealth.ca/article?contentid=2846&language=english#/.

Chapter 3

Strength: When I am Weak, Where is My Strength

…I am the voice of strength.

My size can appear small but is not an indication of my impact. For even in small things, I thrive. I work in and through people. One of my best attributes is I don't discriminate. It doesn't matter to me if you are tall, short, male, female, young, old, or your skin color. I will be there to keep pushing you and keep raising you up. I will be there as your encourager… "You've got this; hold on just a little longer." I am there for you to help others, and I am the voice in your head, never letting your hope fail. I am always rooting for you!

God Does Not Let Go

"So do not fear, for I am with you; do not be dismayed, for I am your God. I will strengthen you and help you; I will uphold you with my righteous right hand."

Isaiah 41:10 NIV

I remember a story, more like a parable, that my dad used to tell, and it has stuck with me over the years. I think it's fairly common, so you may have heard of it.

It's the story of the drowning man:

During a flood, a fellow was stuck on his rooftop and prayed to God for strength and help. Soon a man in a rowboat came by and shouted to the man on the roof, "Jump in; I can save you." The stranded man yelled back, "No, it's OK. I'm praying to God, and He is going to give me strength and save me." So the rowboat went on.

Then a motorboat came by. He yelled as the situation worsened and the water rose, "Jump in; I can save you." To this, the stranded man responded again, "No, it's OK. I'm praying to God, and He is going to give me strength and save me." So the motorboat went on.

62

Then a helicopter came by, and the pilot shouted down, "Grab this rope, and I will lift you to safety." To this, the stranded man responded once again, "No, it's OK. I'm praying to God, and He is going to give me strength and save me." So the helicopter reluctantly flew away.

Soon the water rose above the rooftop, and the man drowned. He went to heaven. He finally got a chance to discuss the whole situation with God, at which point he exclaimed, "I had faith in you that you would give me strength and save me, but you didn't. I don't understand why!"

To this, God replied, "I sent you a rowboat, motorboat, and a helicopter; what more did you expect?"

God sends those around us to help us and maybe bring us to safety. It isn't always in the timing that we plan, and sometimes it is not in the way we expect. However, I trust that God is personally involved in our lives. Our Pastor, Neil White, often says, "I trust that somehow God is in the midst of this." Regardless of our circumstances, Pastor Neil's quote gives me a sense of peace. God never lets us go, even though, at times, we might feel as if we are like the man waiting alone on a rooftop... waiting for a miracle that is on our terms. Perhaps you feel the waters rise around you, waiting for God to come. Maybe you are saying, "No thanks," to the help offered because you think something more is coming, or this isn't quite what you have imagined. I believe God uses others around us (family, friends, church, and therapists) in addition to science and modern medicine to help us. He may have provided those around you as your rowboat or helicopter, saying, "Jump in, I can help." May we recognize when God is giving us strength through using the gifts of others in our lives. It was never intended for us to live in this world alone, and thank God...*we do not have to.*

> **It was never intended for us to live in this world alone, and thank God...*we do not have to.***

To share a bit more personally, in addition to the cancer journeys with my son and husband, the medical community is no stranger to me. I have been a type 1 Diabetic since I was 8 years old and rely on insulin and continuous glucose monitors to manage my health. I am familiar with calculating carbohydrates and managing highs and lows of blood sugar. I wear an insulin pump, and even as a little girl, my parents pushed me and gave me confidence that I never had to be hindered by Diabetes. Never let that hold you back. I went through different phases of my love-hate relationship with Diabetes. There were rebellious times during my teenage years. Still, Diabetes also propelled my first job out of college, working for an amazing company that helps people with Diabetes. I felt a sense of belonging and knew I wasn't alone with Diabetes. When Alex and I were dating (during those teenage and early adult years when I wanted to ignore Diabetes), he was genuinely interested in learning more about Diabetes because it was part of me.

Even when we were 20 years old, he would sometimes drive me to my quarterly endocrinology appointments, a two-hour drive to Denver. I remember it gave us lots of time to talk, laugh, and listen to music in the car and a slight sense of independence. Even then, he was my rock. We would load up in Alex's red Oldsmobile with a bench seat. I liked the bench seat and would scoot over close to him; it was cozy. I also liked that he took an interest in my health and had a passion for healthcare. Alex has committed his professional career to the medical field. In retrospect, we were prepared to frequently go by hospitals and have the healthcare community as our rowboats during his and Sal's cancer treatments.

To reflect on a few historical scientists, I am grateful for their significant impact and contributions to modern medicine. I am grateful for Sir Frederick G Banting, Charles H Best, and John James Rickard Macleod, the creators of insulin over 100 years ago in 1921. I can now face each day, and people with Diabetes can now live fully and not be hindered by the disease[1]. I also reflect and think of the history of chemotherapy. [2] I am grateful for Sidney Farber who studied Childhood Leukemia. These doctors and scientists are truly a gift from God – they are the helicopters with the ropes saying, "hang on, I'll help you." In addition to the many scientists, chemists, and doctors, I encourage anyone struggling with emotional and mental health to also lean on therapists, psychologists, and pastors who can use their gifts to help strengthen us when we need a reminder that we matter. You matter. Your child matters.

So with confidence, I can say God does not let go. Isaiah reminds us time and time again of God walking with us through the mess. *"So do not fear, for I am with you; do not be dismayed, for I am your God. I will strengthen you and help you; I will uphold you with my righteous right hand." Isaiah 41:10 NIV.* What do you see that is missing in this verse? Or, better yet, sometimes I ask myself, what is it that the verse doesn't say. It does not say that God will heal us from every disease. It does not say that we will not have trials and struggles that are sometimes chronic and will be with us for the rest of our lives. Maybe you are not facing a physical struggle but a relational struggle. Perhaps it is a failed relationship or an addiction. None of us are immune to suffering. However, God reminds us that He is with us and will strengthen us to face the storms ahead, whether He sends motorboats, helicopters, or sometimes it takes the form of the uniquely gifted healthcare community.

The Faith of a Child

"As he went along, he saw a man blind from birth. His disciples asked him, "Rabbi, who sinned, this man or his parents, that he was born blind?" "Neither this man nor his parents sinned," said Jesus, "but this happened so that the work of God might be displayed in his life."

John 9:1-3 NIV

In the verse above, we are brought into an intimate moment with a family that meets Jesus, and the disciples ask what we all ask when a child is blind, deaf...*or has cancer*. When the world seems so unkind and unfair, we want to find the cause and effect. We want to blame ourselves or maybe even those around us. Have you ever been there? I remember thinking many times, "God, what happened? Was this my fault? Did I do something?" I remember pouring over the research on what causes childhood cancer and trying to grasp onto something that would maybe provide an answer because then I would as least know...*why*. I can almost reply to this same story plot in my own head but with a modern twist. It would go something like this...

> **"God, what happened? Was this my fault? Did I do something?"**

...As we went along, I saw my child with cancer. I asked Jesus, "But, Why God? Who sinned? Did I do something wrong? Did we eat the wrong food–maybe it was McDonald's or Chick-Fil-A? Did I sin? Maybe it's because I gave him formula? Is it because I bought non-brand name baby food and fed that to him when he was 6 months old?" The list keeps going on in my head, and I replay every parenting decision and purchase I made.

Did I use the wrong sunscreen? Maybe I was cleaning with the wrong cleaning supplies? Or perhaps it was that I cleaned too much. (If you know me, I hate cleaning, so there is no way I'd be cleaning too much. But it still didn't stop the ludicrous thought from popping in my head). Was it our detergent? I wonder if it's because I didn't check for BPA's until he was older. Wait, I know what it is for sure...did Alex do something to cause this? (Small joke because it's easy to blame the husband). It will literally make your mind go crazy.

...And then the peace that passes all understanding calms our hearts and minds. God answers me, *"My precious daughter, you did nothing to cause this, so don't carry the blame and shame. Don't worry; My Work will be displayed in your child's life. Their life matters to me. They are my child too. Don't worry; I am still in control."*

I finally realized I will never know "why" explained in a way that makes sense to me. I had to surrender and learn there is an unknown side of God, but I still trust He is in the midst of this with us. He is in the midst of this with you, too...*even if you are now thoroughly convinced you used the wrong sunscreen...*take a breath; you did nothing wrong for your child to get cancer.

69

As I reflect further on how God has used this to shape Sal's faith, I see the beautiful trust and faith of a child who simply hopes and sees God's goodness in all things. I remember the times Sal and I often played thumb war or "I spy with my little eye" during the many hospital stays or while we waited in the waiting room. There is a lot of waiting time during the Leukemia journey. Life slows, and priorities come into focus.

I will never know "why" explained in a way that makes sense to me.

One particular day while I was home with Sal during one of the more aggressive times of chemo, we went outside to sit on the porch for a few minutes. Sal had his precious bald head, and his skin was pale. His face still had joy, but his physical features were changing. I remember seeing his eyes had dark circles. He was too tired to play, and his body was extremely worn out. There was no way we'd be able to go for even a short walk around our neighborhood, so we decided to sit on the front step outside our house and just get some fresh air.

Sal said, "Hey Mom, Do you want to play, 'I spy with my little eye,' with me?"

To be honest, I was tired, but I went along with it.

Sal: "Ok, great, I get to start. I spy with my little eye something that starts with G."

Me: I looked around and the first thing that caught my eye I say, "Grass."

Sal: "Nope," he said with a huge grin.

Me: Hmm, what else, I think to myself. Got it, I said, "Green leaves."

Sal: "Nope"

Me: "Ok, I am stumped; I give up."

Sal: "God's glory all around…don't you see it, mom?"

Wow, I thought. Sal has so much wisdom and faith… the faith of a child. He sees so clearly. If I am honest with myself, I couldn't see God's glory at that moment…and if I am really being honest, I wasn't looking for God's glory either. I was just wishing and praying for this to be over.

This intimate moment brought me strength and encouragement to keep pressing forward. If my brave warrior, whose body is going through an intense battle, can look at the world around and innocently see God's glory, then the work of God is being displayed, and I can have peace knowing God is in control. A reminder of Jesus' words, *"that the work of God might be displayed in his life." John 9:1-3.* The faith of a child can teach us so much.

So next time you step outside and look around, I encourage you to play a little game with yourself...I spy with my little eye something that starts with G...*do you see it?*

When the unexpected happens again (Alex's cancer diagnosis)

"I have made you and I will carry you; I will sustain you and I will rescue you."

Isaiah 46:4 NIV

Once you hear "Your child has cancer," from that moment on, very few things in life can send a shock wave to your core like those words...*except when you hear them again.* This time it was a slightly different ring; it was more vague and unsure. The doctor said, *"It might be cancer."* Huh? Did I hear that right? What does that even mean? Below is an excerpt from my journal.

Journal Entry March 1, 2020

It's been about a month since we have known. Alex had significant pain and went to the ER. Through a CT scan, they found a mass on his pancreas. We suddenly got thrust into a world of "pancreatic cancer." What is this disease? Does he have it? How is this the same or different from leukemia? Through several different doctors and healthcare providers and different imaging (MRI, multiple CTs)...we now have more information. It is about 5 cm on the tail of the pancreas. The best option is to surgically remove the tumor, along with the tail of the pancreas, spleen, and lymph nodes. He will be hospitalized for several days, and then we'll know the pathology and if he will need chemo. The doctor believes it to be pancreatic neuroendocrine cancer. Slow growing cancer and far better prognosis. We feel hopeful and encouraged. And so we wait until we know. The surgery date is March 12. And so we wait, we trust, we hope, and we pray.

My heart reached out in prayer to the one who knows the answers...

I leveled with God..."I need to know. Is it cancer?"

Yahweh's gentle nudge, "Yes, get ready...I have made you and I will carry you; I will sustain you and I will rescue you." Isaiah 46:4 NIV

73

The anticipation leading up to surgery is one of the hardest things to keep tame. Life still moves on and work continues even though the first thought of the day and the last thought revolves around counting down the days until the surgery and preparing everything there is to prepare in advance. I already felt like I was dealing with an impossible situation with Sal's diagnosis and now Alex. Cancer does not exempt you from other challenges that emerge in life. The Lord promises us He will "carry, sustain, and rescue" us when the monster stares us down and looks overwhelming.

The word "might be" is one of the scariest thoughts. I remember weeping for Sal because I didn't know the intimate details of the cancer journey. The unknown was extremely frightening, but now cancer is no longer unknown to our family. I weep now because I now know what this could mean...I know what the "might be" reality feels like. In those raw and soul-gripping moments, we are reminded time and time again of God's promises. The creator of the universe intimately

> **Cancer does not exempt you from other challenges that emerge in life.**

tells us he will carry, sustain, and rescue us. We don't have to go it alone. God is our strength.

Fast forward now to March 12, 2020; it was about 4:45 pm in the waiting room. Alex had gone into surgery several hours earlier. He was ready for this next step. He had a sense of peace within him. My mom was at our house staying with Sal. I had spoken to them both earlier in the day, and Sal sounded happy. The TV in the waiting room was on, and the only news coverage was about a new virus spreading around the world called Coronavirus. Something odd was going on globally. The word "pandemic" was being used, but none of us knew what that meant yet. I was the only person in the waiting room by this time as slowly, one by one, the other care-givers trickled out. The waiting room was almost a perfect square followed by a hallway, and it had enough chairs to probably fit at least 25-30 people. The front desk lady was not chatty and was wrapping up for the day. I probably gave off all the non-verbal cues of "not interested in talking," too, so we avoided eye contact. I got up and walked down the other side of the hallway. The hospital was immaculate and had bright lights with older, darker blue upholstery chairs and wooden frames.

By the time I got back from the hallway, the TV was off, and the front desk lady had gone home for the night. I sat by a window, and the hallway was empty and still. I was alone.

I waited and waited. Checking my cell phone, it was now about 6:15 pm; the surgery had gone long...about an hour over. It felt like forever. The nurse in the surgery had called me a couple of hours earlier and said everything was going fine, but it would take a bit longer. I wasn't sure what that meant, but I held onto the hope in the words "everything was going fine." It was dark outside.

Then, I heard the movement of feet walking. The surgeon came right up to me with optimism in the air. He said with pride and a grin as he clenched his fist high in the air in a victorious way, "I got it all. The margins are clean. I got it all! Pathology is running more tests, and they believe it is Stage I Pancreatic Neuroendocrine Cancer, just as I expected. We got it early; he's lucky. He is doing well. He is in recovery, and you can see him in about 20 minutes. I'll be back tomorrow during rounds to check on him. He's going to be ok." The surgeon briskly walked away with confidence in his step while giving a gentle touch on my shoulder. Those words brought immense relief. Such wonderful news! I smiled with joy. He left, and I was alone again in the waiting room. But this time, I didn't feel lonely. There was rejoicing!

God's promises in Isaiah are an anchor and a source of strength. What a relief! I don't have to rely on my own strength and don't have to rely on my own emotions. God promises He will carry us through, He will sustain us as we patiently wait alone, and ultimately, we know our rescue is coming.

Alex got settled into the hospital room, and I was next to him with my blankets from home and my hospital couch bed set up (I was starting to get used to these hospital bed setups). Alex was attached to lots of tubes and lots of machines. (Yes, those same beeping machines like the ones at Children's Hospital). Even among all that noise, I rested that night knowing the cancer is removed, knowing God carries us, sustains us, and rescues us.

That night was a moment of peace to treasure... *however*, within the next 24 hours, Alex spiked a fever and an infection started. Little did we know what the next 6 months would bring as the storm was cunningly waiting for him around the corner.

Friendship in unforeseen and abundant ways

"A friend loves at all times."

Proverbs 17:17 NIV

Sal was in 2nd grade attending partially a Montessori school when he was able to be in school. He also spent many months homeschooled by my mom, who graciously and sacrificially became his teacher. As we were gearing up for him to go into a phase called Delayed Intensification, the hospital gave us a video that he could share with his classmates about what to expect and some educational materials on Leukemia. Delayed Intensification is a re-induction phase that gives intense chemotherapy before the maintenance phase starts to share more about the phases. Sal would be quarantined for most of Delayed Intensification because the plan is to bottom out the immune system to kill any residual Leukemia cells that might still be hiding.[3] Delayed Intensification is eight weeks, and a variety of aggressive chemotherapies are given both at the hospital through his port and chemotherapy pills. Alex and I were both trained on giving him injection shots as well. Sal's body would need to fight to survive.

We arranged with Sal's 2nd-grade teacher to have a designated time where the kids could watch the video and ask some questions. I was grateful for this resource from the hospital as Sal would return to school in a few months, and his physical features would look different. He likely would not have hair and may be very weak and thin.

We watched the video and then opened up for a few questions from the class. One little boy, who I will never forget, raised his hand like he had something crucial to say. The teacher motioned for him to share, and he looked at Sal with the most caring and compassionate human eyes, "Sal, when you come back, and you are too weak to carry your backpack; don't you worry, I can carry both our backpacks." *Wow, I thought…the truest form of empathy.*

"…don't you worry, I can carry both our backpacks."

The class quickly moved on to other questions, but this stuck with me. This little boy got it. He gets it, what we sometimes, as adults, forget. He knew what it was to be a friend. "A friend loves at all times…" Proverbs 17:17a NIV Who are those in your life who, when you got tired, volunteered to help carry the load? Even as adults, we have versions of our backpacks that we carry. We have the burdens of life, guilt, and shame of something in the past. Even the backpack of anxiety of our worst fears playing out in our heads. Yet, these burdens feel so real. Those around us help us indeed carry our "backpacks."

There is a quote that I resonate with from George Washington Carver. To provide some context on George Washing Carver, he was born into slavery and then became one of the most prominent scientists and inventors using one of our typical household food items... peanuts.[4] George Washington Carver knew first-hand what it was to encounter adversity and experienced both the beauty and ugliness of humanity. His quote speaks of the empathy of humanity.

"How far you go in life depends on your being tender with the young, compassionate with the aged, sympathetic to the striving and tolerant of the weak and the strong, because someday in life, you will have been all of these."

– George Washington Carver[5]

During our Leukemia journey, we were weak and needed help. The Lord provided people who were praying for us, helping with meals, helping with cleaning, and general support because our tender young child was facing an enemy. We had people who were patient with us when life became very inward-focused on our family. I had a neighbor who would drop off a meal once a week at the house for over a year. She did not need recognition or glory. She didn't even stay and chat because she knew we were exhausted, and I didn't have the energy for small talk. She simply dropped it off every Wednesday and sent a quick text, "Dinner is on the porch." I could never repay her for her commitment and being a constant friend. Someone who indeed carried our "backpack."

Out of the generosity of their hearts, I had several co-workers who gave gifts for Sal, sent me cards of encouragement, and UberEats gift cards for our family because we needed help. They stepped up for me and "carried my backpack" at work when I needed to be away. My boss gave me grace and flexibility so I could continue my career while also focusing on my family. One of my close co-workers was always a phone call away and always made the time to talk when I needed it. She lived in Florida; however, distance didn't stop her from reaching and helping in a close way. She gathered our team, and they pooled their resources together. Throughout the three-plus years of Sal's cancer journey, they would occasionally send him gifts and encouragements for our brave warrior. They seemed to come on a random day and were such a pleasant surprise! Every time a package would arrive, the timing was impeccable. It always came during a week when we needed a lift, and it brought a smile to Sal's face. They carried my burdens and supported us when we needed them. I will never forget my co-workers who stepped up in more ways than I could have ever expected.

And lastly, my sister-in-law, Christie, provided tremendous support and was someone who metaphorically carried my backpack. Christie is Alex's older sister. She has blond hair and an athletic build. Christie, her husband Mark, and their two girls live in Wyoming; they love the outdoors and everything about Wyoming. Christie traveled from Wyoming several times to see Sal in the hospital and help with anything I needed help with. I remember when she came out to Texas because Sal had been in the hospital for several weeks. I don't think I had even stepped outside for several days because I didn't want to leave Sal's side. She must have noticed that I needed a break, even if I was trying to appear strong to those around me. She secretly talked to the nurses and found a place to take me out for a quick hour and get a pedicure. Alex stayed with Sal, and she surprised me and just said with a confident smile, "Come on, I made the appointment; we're getting pedicures today." I didn't want to disappoint her. If she had asked me ahead of time, I would have come up with a reason not to go. She probably knew this as well, so she just went ahead and scheduled it. She knew I needed to get fresh air and clear my head. She knew I needed a change of scenery. And, she was right! I came back with sparkling pink toes, and I felt refreshed. It sure does bring a smile to your face when you're in the hospital room, and you get to look down and see your toes with a bright and beautiful color. It makes you feel pretty, even if your feet are the only thing that feels bright during those long dark days in the hospital. I am forever grateful for my sister-in-law, Christie.

We were grateful for those who came to our aid.

On the flip side, during the cancer journey, the inner circle of friends can sometimes become small. There are many reasons why and sometimes, in the cancer community, there is a common saying, "You'll know who your friends are." Which implies judgment. Our inner circle became small, too; however, some of it was our own choice. Before cancer, I had some very close friends who were not part of the inner circle. But I have realized, as the proverb reminds us, "A friend loves at all times." Proverb 17:17 NIV Not every friend is meant to walk intimately with you on this journey...and that is ok. They are still friends, those before and after cancer, and as George Washington Carver says above...be *compassionate, sympathetic, and tolerant* both for those who have chosen to become part of the inner circle and those friends or family members who stayed on the sidelines. It's ok; there is a role for both. Even in the unexpected disappointments of some friends who you expected to show up more, it's ok. You will also see the unexpected kindness and generosity of others that have now become part of the inner circle as it is an honor for them that is not necessarily meant for the masses.

So, as we look at strength. I encourage you to allow others to carry your "backpack" when needed. Be looking out for those who might need someone to take their "backpack" as their world now appears cruel, and they need relief from the weight of it all. Reflect on those unexpected moments where humanity showed the grace of Jesus through compassion, sympathy, and tolerance.

Who is lifting up your arms?

"As long as Moses held up his hands, the Israelites were winning, but whenever he lowered his hands, the Amalekites were winning. When Moses' hand grew tired, they took a stone and put it under so he sat on it. Aaron and Hur held up his hands – one on one side, one on the other side – so that his hands remained steady till sunset"

Exodus 17: 11-13 NIV

Can you see the image? Moses, Aaron, and Hur are on a mountain top while Joshua and the Israelites fight the battle in the valley. Moses has the staff of God in his hands. As long as his arms are raised, his people are winning. To be candid, this story is just kind of bizarre and weird yet shows us time and time again about a loving God who never intended for us to fight our battles on our own. We need each other for support. We need each other to lift our arms.

I have a small request, maybe just a simple dare for you to see if you can do it. (I've tried, and I can't, but I want to see

85

how you do). Just during this one section, as you read, raise one of your hands up above your head and keep it there. How long does it take you for your arm to get tired? Maybe a couple of minutes? Perhaps you can go longer? Your arm, at some point, will start to burn, and you will need to find some relief. Don't put it down yet; keep your arm up.

I love this story because no matter how strong we think we are, there is a limit, and then we need the strength of others. I had two people holding up my arms while Alex and Sal fought their battle. You, too, will have one or two people on your journey who you can trust to be there and ready to give you a seat and hold the weight towards victory. Maybe even as you read this, you are one of the people who are needed to help raise someone else's arms and give additional strength. Just checking, is your arm still up? How is it going? (Ok, my point is made, you can put your arm down now at any time).

We need each other for support. We need each other to lift our arms.

My sister, Mandy, was the first person who held up my arms when I got tired and needed rest.. My sister was my

"Anchor." She didn't always have to be in the boat with us, but she was on the entire journey. She was grounded and did not sway. I called her often with the ups and downs, and she was solid. She had an "Assignment" and knew God uniquely called her for a purpose. Nothing was off-limits between us, and there was no judgment. She knew Sal was being cared for and provided with many things, so although she continued to be a supportive aunt, she knew her primary "Assignment" was support for me. My big sister was assigned as my anchor! Lastly, she was an "Ambassador." An Ambassador is someone working for the government, but she was an "Ambassador" for Christ in this case. I know she was praying for our family and me. I know her heart was also pierced when I had a hard day. She could adjust quickly to my mood at the moment to lighten the vibe when I just wanted to talk about something…just anything other than cancer. Just something normal…I didn't care, anything at all… "So, tell me, what's going on with you? What's on sale at Costco?"

I remember during the COVID-19 quarantine when we couldn't be close and had to social distance. I craved my sister being near us and missed being able to hug her.

Sal and her three children go to the same school, so while Sal was doing virtual school, we had a folder that they would drop off at our house with his schoolwork at the beginning of the week. Then at the end of the week we would drop it off at their house to return to Sal's teacher for grading.

One evening, it was really late at night, and we somehow forgot to drop the folder off, and we needed to get it to her house. Additionally, Sal had a lumbar puncture and was home resting. It was heartbreaking to see his pain and discomfort. It was a hard day. Alex was also recovering which was going ok but slow. It was very late at night; while the family was sleeping, I texted Mandy and said, "I am coming with the folder; sorry it is so late, I can stick it in your garage." As I pulled up to her dark house, I saw her on their outdoor patio bench in the small glimmer of her porch light. She got my text and was there, just waiting to see me. I got out of the car, and she walked toward me; I couldn't hold it back. I ran to her with wide arms. She wrapped her arms around me and gave me one of the most uplifting hugs as I cried and yelled, "I hate this! I hate this!" She just held me until the wave of emotion passed. She was figuratively holding up my arms when I needed strength.

My mom was the second person by my side, holding up my arms. From the moment of Sal's diagnosis, she committed to helping us. The words I used to describe my mom are "servant's heart." She served in many ways. She lived with us periodically throughout Sal's treatment and filled any gap I needed. She cooked, cleaned, and served us unrelentingly even during her grief about my Dad's death. She showed me the true definition of "sacrificial love," and I know she put her own needs on hold while caring for us.

One of my mom's roles she quickly slid into is that she became Sal's teacher when he needed to be home-schooled. She said she always wanted to be a teacher, and who would have thought that as a retired grandma, God still had work for her to do. It's a good reminder that we are never too old to do God's work. Sal enjoyed "Bamma" (the name he calls my mom) as his teacher. Mom taught the basics...math, vocabulary, reading, etc. She also took on a few extra curriculums; she was his PE teacher! Wow, it was fun to see them play our unique version of baseball/whiffle ball in the backyard when Sal was feeling well enough to go outside. Mom was always good about making us go outside and get fresh air each day. She taught Sal how to read a clock and about commerce so he could earn some money. I will never forget the day I walked out of my office, and mom had set up all of Sal's stuffed animals, spreading them across the living room. They were pretending Sal was the owner of a pet shop. She was purchasing pets and pet accessories from him. Mom had a handful of nickels and quarters Sal "earned" through his pet shop that he was able to keep. Wow, did he feel rich that day! In fact, it was a day we all felt rich with lots of smiles and laughter. In more ways than one, my mom was by my side holding my arms up when the weight was too heavy.

In more ways than one, my mom was by my side holding my arms up when the weight was too heavy.

If you are reading right now and having one of those "hard days," you know I am talking about those days; I understand what you are going through. I know the complete exhaustion and tiredness that sleep won't even cure. Today, my prayer is that this gives you the strength to help lift your arms. When life is heavy, remember Victory Is Ahead.

Practical Tip – Source of Strength

Here are a few quotes for others who have endured the journey of childhood cancer and their advice to other caregivers about a source of strength and support during treatment. This section is intended to give you some alternate perspectives and show you that there are different choices that families and caretakers make that are best for their family circumstances. Before doing anything drastic, consider all your options for support and have confidence that you are doing the best thing you can for your child.

> "I quit my job and just focused on our son with cancer. This was the best decision for us and our family. I just couldn't see myself doing anything else" (Mom of a son with cancer)

> "I took FMLA (Family Medical Leave Act) medical leave for a period of time during the most aggressive chemo months and then returned to work. My employer was not always flexible but I was able

to navigate as best as I could because I needed to keep my job for the medical benefits" (Dad of a son with cancer)

"I immediately used my PTO (Paid Time Off) and then took an extended leave of absence. After a couple of months, I partnered with my boss for flexibility so I could keep working. My work provided me a sense of stability when life felt out of control" (Mom of a son who had cancer)

"It's all major." (Oncologist stated when asked what parts of the journey are hardest)

"Share the Care! I knew I was along for the long haul. I had a special role and knew that this would be a marathon. One piece of advice to other caregivers is when new people step in to help in a variety of ways, it's ok to share the care. It doesn't mean you aren't doing something you should do, it's ok for them to support those going through cancer on the frontlines too in their own way. Allow yourself to Share the Care." (My sister)

"You can make grief your friend or you can make grief your enemy." (My mom)

"It's been a topsy-turvy year. Good thing God can do somersaults while he holds us in his arms" (My Mom)

"We got connected with our social worker at the hospital who provided several financial resources for us and we worked with the hospital towards a payment plan due to some of the larger medical bills. The social worker also put us in touch with the Make-a-Wish organization that gave my daughter something to look forward to." (Mom of a daughter who had cancer)

Notes

1   "The History of a Wonderful Thing We Call Insulin," American Diabetes Association, Updated July 1, 2019 https://www.diabetes.org/blog/history-wonderful-thing-we-call-insulin.

2   Siddhartha Mukherjee, *The Emperor of All Maladies: A Biography of Cancer* (United Stated, 2010).

3   "Treatments for Childhood ALL," Canadian Cancer Society, accessed on January 28, 2022, https://cancer.ca/en/cancer-information/cancer-types/leukemia-childhood/treatment/acute-lymphocytic-leukemia-all.

4   "George Washing Carver," *Biography*, updated on April 27, 2017, https://www.biography.com/scientist/george-washington-carver.

5   "George Washington Carver Quotes and Sayings – Page 1," *Inspiring Quotes*, accessed on January 28, 2022, https://www.inspiringquotes.us/author/4029-george-washington-carver#:~:text=%E2%80%9CHow%20far%20you%20go%20in,have%20been%20all%20of%20these.%E2%80%9D.

Chapter 4

Security: Nothing about this is Comfortable

…I am the voice of security along with my twin named control.
We go hand and hand – security and control. When one of us
rises up, the other reacts. When one of us tanks to a low point,
the other twin will overcompensate. Most people don't notice
us when life is calm and composed. When there is a balance of
security and life is in control, we barely get attention. But in
crisis, boy oh boy…control just goes off the handle unchecked.
And me, well, I either grow timid and scared, or I can go big
and bold trying to grasp onto something that will be safe. We
may get misbranded as irritability, feelings of inadequacy,
jealousy, perfectionism, and unhealthy comparison. My twin
and I are somewhat unpredictable and can get into your head.
But don't worry, somehow faith has a way of showing up and
eventually calms the storm.

God, Our Comforter, has a Plan

"For I know the plans I have for you, declare the Lord. Plans to prosper you and not to harm you. Plans to give you hope and a future."

Jeremiah 29:11 NIV

Have you ever had something break, and it seemed like a simple fix at first, but it grew and grew and was anything but simple? Perhaps a home project or car problems? Those little annoyances and frustrations in life seem to jump out right at the worst time!

During the COVID-19 quarantine in February of 2021, our dishwasher broke. This was a relatively new dishwasher, only about 2 years old. So, my first frustration and what I was thinking in my head was, "We just bought this thing, and it broke already!" It was still under warranty, so I called the warranty company. They had the first dishwasher repairman come out, one of the rudest people I have ever encountered. This resulted in him being asked to leave and me calling the company back for a new repairman. He didn't fix it and just caused more frustration. Then a second appointment was made, and the repairman never showed up. Well, that's just great. The third time was a charm, right? Six weeks had now gone by, and we were hand washing dishes. Every evening I looked at my dishwasher and the constant reminder that this stupid thing was broken.

The third repairman was scheduled to come, so I was waiting that day to have someone finally fix it! I was upstairs working in my office as my job had moved permanently to work from home due to COVID-19. Sal was across the hallway doing digital school as he was still quarantined due to his immune system. My mom was at the house with us as she came during quarantine to help with many things.

Suddenly, there is a knock at the door. My office window is upstairs and overlooks the front of our house, so I see every car that drives down our street. There was no car, and no one drove by. "Huh, that's weird." I think to myself. My mom let the gentleman in; he was short in stature with dark hair. But the thing I noticed most was his smile. Joy was seeping out of this man. He had on a shirt with the warranty company's name, and he said, "I'm here for the dishwasher." "Oh, great!" I say to myself. "Finally, let's get this thing fixed."

I show the repairman into the kitchen, and he begins to set down his tools and work on the dishwasher. Within a few minutes, he begins to speak to my mom, and she shares with him that her grandson, Sal, is doing digital school online because he has Leukemia. He then calmly and gently said to me, "Don't worry, everything is going to be ok with your son." An unexplainable peace settles over me. I shared more about our situation with him, and he began to share that he is a believer. He has two children, and he shares a testimony about God healing one of them. The whole time he is working on the dishwasher, he ministers to us and reminds us of God's amazing healing and to trust the plan. *"For I know the plans I have for you, declare the Lord. Plans to prosper you and not to harm you. Plans to give you hope and a future." Jeremiah 29:11 NIV. Now* get this, as he wrapped up, he said, "Well, I wasn't able to fix your dishwasher. A replacement part will be here in a couple of weeks, and someone else will come and fix it." And then, I will never forget his final words as he left. He said, "This is small stuff for God. Your son will be healed. Don't worry, everything will be ok." Again, this unexplainable peace and joy overcame me. He prayed out loud for my son.

A peace that passes all understanding. I wasn't even mad that our dishwasher still wasn't fixed, but I felt a larger-than-life flame of HOPE, and that victory was around the corner. The finish line was in sight! Amen!

He left and walked out the door. I still don't recall seeing his truck or car, and not quite sure where he went. Afterward, I asked my mom, "Did you see his car?" She said no. I said, "Who was that man?" And she said, "A messenger from God." An affirmation of HOPE! We speculated that he was an angel in disguise or just a man on a mission from God. Regardless of who he was, he was a messenger that brought comfort and peace to trust in God's plan.

Several weeks later, right after Easter, a fourth repairman did come and finally fixed the dishwasher! Yay!!! We joked as it was broken the entire time during lent. Unknowingly, I gave up using my dishwasher for lent.

Maybe you are the messenger God is sending to others to remind them of Jeremiah 29:11 *"For I know the plans I have for you, declare the Lord. Plans to prosper you and not to harm you. Plans to give you hope and a future." Or, maybe you needed to hear these words today.* Or, perhaps, you might have a messenger at your door.

God Never Wastes Anything

"What you have meant for evil; God meant for Good"

Genesis 50:20 NLT

I am now thoroughly convinced that God hears every conversation, even the smallest voices. My sister-in-law, Heather, came to help us for a few days during one of the phases called Consolidation. Consolidation was the second phase in our journey and can typically last for several months. This phase further reduces the number of leukemia cells still in the body, and different chemotherapies are used to help prevent the remaining leukemia cells from developing resistance.[1]

To set the stage and give a little more context, I am the youngest of four children in my family, and there is a 12-year difference between my oldest brother and me. My oldest brother, Steve, met Heather in High School when they were, 16 so quite literally, she has known me since I was 4 years old. Our family is close even though my two older brothers and their families live far away. (And trust me, I've tried to convince them all to move to Texas, but they seem to enjoy their own home states). Steve, Heather, and their family live in Colorado, and

Heather generously came to stay with us during one of Sal's lumbar puncture weeks when he was on a heavy dose of chemo and steroids. Steroid weeks were always the most challenging and exhausting.

Heather has always been tall and lean, with slightly longer than shoulder-length hair that is wavy. Heather has a gift of making others feel comfortable around her, and she is one of the people in my life who is easy to talk to and she laughs often. While Heather was helping us at our house, we had a conversation with Sal regarding birthstones. He started to read about gems and stones and really studied rocks, especially learning the birthstones. A friend had sent him a box of different gems and a book. It's incredible to see how rocks were formed and the gems' beauty.

Sal was born in February, so his birthstone is a gorgeous purple Amethyst. We saw many pictures of Amethyst and loved the magnificent eggplant and purple shades as they shine. He was begging to have his own genuine amethyst as the start of his first rock collection since the original kit of gems did not have an Amethyst in it. I think he asked us to buy him an Amethyst every day for a week straight...he was persistent.

On one particular day, as the conversation unfolded, we went around and shared what each person had as their birthstone. I was proud to have Opal for October. Any October birthdays out there? We then got to Heather, who was a December baby. She bluntly says, "I gotta be honest, I hate my birthstone. I just don't like the color Turquoise." Sal immediately looked at her with shock and was thoroughly insulted by what she said. He takes his hand up slightly to his mouth and whispers over to her, and very pointedly says, "Aunt Heather, don't say that!" We are both confused now, and I try and quickly recall if Heather said something inappropriate or perhaps a bad word. My brain is trying to figure out why he is so offended by her statement. And then he confidently points up, still whispering, and says, "Don't say that too loudly; it's Jesus' birthstone, and he'll hear you." Oh, I see now. He was boldly standing up for Jesus, and he was not going to let anyone talk badly about Jesus' birthstone. I will be candid; I had never thought about Jesus having a birthstone, have you? Through Sal's eyes, Jesus is tangible and there with us, just as if Jesus was physically sitting next to us on the couch. Of course, Jesus would have a birthstone of his own; everyone has a birthstone, right? Sal's tangible faith provides comfort for us all.

As I reflect, that was a week meant to be hard, full of pain and suffering due to the chemo. However, Genesis 50:20 reminds us, *"What is meant for Evil, God meant for Good."* We got to cherish and reflect on each of our own birthstones and the preciousness of each gem. Curious about your thoughts on your own birthstone. Do you like your birthstone? Maybe you have a gorgeous purple Amethyst like Sal, or perhaps you have the cherished Diamond for April, or an Emerald for May. Alex has Topaz for November. Do you wish it was different? Or, better yet, are you one of the lucky people who share their birthstone with Jesus?

Now, get this! Sal got a package in the mail a few days later: an educational kit about random countries. Inside the box was also a genuine Amethyst. There was no note indicating who it was from. I asked Heather if she sent it as that would be the most logical person because of our recent conversation. She said, "Nope." We discovered it was from another extended family member who had no way of knowing we were talking about birthstones and had no way of knowing what the kit would have inside.

Amazing…Sal got his Amethyst.

I know what you might be thinking; that's just a coincidence…what's the big deal? Maybe God orchestrated a way for Sal to receive an Amethyst as a "God wink," saying, "thanks for sticking up for my birthstone, buddy." It was so personal to Sal, so we are reminded, *"What was meant for evil, God meant for Good."*

> **God hears the tiniest conversations, and then He delivers in an extraordinarily comforting and wowed way.**

God hears the tiniest conversations, and then He delivers in an extraordinarily comforting and wowed way. A great reminder that God never wastes anything…even our most inconsequential conversations about silly rocks.

You are not Alone: COVID-19

"Have I not commanded you? Be strong and courageous. Do not be afraid; do not be discouraged, for the Lord your God will be with you wherever you go."

Joshua 1:9 NIV

The statistics on Pancreatic Cancer are anything but comforting. It's known as the silent killer.[2] We initially had some hope and found comfort in Alex's prognosis. He was diagnosed with Pancreatic Neuroendocrine Cancer, which has a far better prognosis. There is roughly a 54% survival rate for more than five years (All SEER stages combined). Also, there was comfort in the staging. He was Stage 1, which means the cancer is localized and has not spread to other parts of the body, with an even better prognosis of 93% survival rate.[3] The only solution was to surgically remove it; otherwise, it would spread. It seems hopeful and comforting from one perspective; however, it was also shared with us that about 5% of patients can get an infection and the risks of relapse.

At first, I was drawn to statistics and wanted to find out more research. It actually drove me a bit crazy because no matter how the numbers add up, it statistically never gives full assurance and comfort. Reflect and think about the last time you were shared a statistic by a doctor regarding your health or a family member. Did it bring you comfort or more uncertainty? Alex and I stopped leaning on the statistics as our comfort early into his journey. It's a vicious cycle of wanting to know more and feeling secure in the numbers, but ultimately, there is no security. If you or someone you know is newly diagnosed, I don't want to discount statistics altogether . If this is something that brings you a level of sanity, please do what you need and is necessary for you to be educated. However, we have found that the statistics are not our comfort in times of trouble. We have a loving God in the scripture who repeatedly encouraged Joshua and encourages us to *"Be Strong and Courageous, do not be terrified. For the Lord, our God goes with you wherever you go."* Joshua 1:9

Alex and I have a funny saying (or not-so-funny saying, depending on how you look at it), and, goodness, did it ever come true for us. It basically goes like this...It doesn't matter if that statistics or number of probability is 1%, 20%, or 75%; if you end up with it, well, then it's 100% for you. The statistic doesn't matter on a personal level...it's either 0% or 100%. It either happened to you, or it didn't. Although statistics can attempt to give some type of hope, to be perfectly candid, there is no such thing as comforting cancer statistics. It always leaves room for that one small chance of relapse, that

> **There is no such thing as comforting cancer statistics.**

less than 5% of something to go wrong, that tiny percentage of something that is just unexplainable.

Alex got an initial infection and was hospitalized for about a week longer than expected after his distal pancreatectomy surgery (Ironically, according to the statistics, he had a less than 5% chance of getting an infection at that time). He was on many antibiotics and multiple drains for the infection that continued to spread and would not subside. Alex was in immense pain, and the recovery was slow. Even after coming home, he continued to spike fevers, and he went back and forth to the hospital for multiple lengthy stays over four months. It was a complete roller coaster and utterly exhausting going back and forth to the hospital. Also, another complexity was added to our household since he had an infection. Alex had to stay separated from Sal at the house as Sal was immune-compromised. Alex had to say quarantined in one room. My mom was there to help as we were in a constant state of cleaning and disinfecting. There was little physical touch and play in our household. I remember being constantly in fear; fear of infection, fear of getting COVID-19, fear Alex would get Sal sick, fear that Sal would get Alex sick, fear that I would get sick, and fear that my mom would get sick. The list just went on and on. I was afraid of sickness.

I remember one time feeling very alone but looking back now, I know God was with me. One evening late at night, Alex spiked a high fever to 102.7. We called the doctor-on-call, and they directed us to go to the ER. We knew he would be hospitalized as they continued to struggle to find the source of his infection. COVID-19 turned the world upside down, and I was not allowed to be with Alex in the hospital. As many of you reading this book know, you may have experienced a similar situation because of the no visitor policy at many hospitals.

I dropped Alex off at the ER outside. There were big signs that only the patient was allowed in as he slowly hobbled inside. I saw a nurse check his temperature at the door. I wanted more than anything to jump out of the car and run into the hospital with him, but I couldn't. I just sat there and waited in my car for several minutes, thinking with every fiber in my being that this felt wrong. I should be next to him. I should be able to advocate for him and explain to them what is wrong. I should be by his side in sickness and health. No matter how hard I tried, wished, and pleaded...the hospital would not allow me in. I couldn't be there next to him. He was alone in the hospital, and his body was fighting an intense infection. I felt alone. I remembered Joshua 1:9, *"The Lord your God is with you wherever you go."* The Lord was not only with me, but He was also with Alex. I could not physically be by Alex's side, but I trusted and hoped in the unseen One. A loving God was sitting next to me in the car as life turned cloudy, and it felt like the storm was never-ending. A loving God was also sitting next to Alex through his suffering. And a loving God is sitting next to you right now as you face trials and struggles.

And a loving God is sitting next to you right now as you face trials and struggles.

That evening, I just couldn't drive away. I just sat in my car staring at the doors of the hospital. I must have looked like a crazy person with my hair in a thrown-together bun, my glasses were on as it was too late to put back in my contacts, and a worn-out T-shirt. I am sure my look said it all "Crazy Wife, Right Here!" After several minutes the same nurse who took Alex's temperature came outside to the car and kindly ushered for me to roll down the window. In such a comforting voice, she said, "You can go now; we will take good care of him." I can only imagine what she was thinking. I said "thanks" in a meek voice and felt embarrassed, but I just didn't know what else to do. Somehow staring at the hospital doors helped me feel closer to Alex, who was sitting inside those walls. I cried as I drove home that night. I wonder how many wives, husbands, moms, and dads she had to say that to that night, "You can go now; we'll take good care of them." She was giving me and any others she had to tell that night comfort and assurance to drive away when our loved one was inside the hospital walls separated from us when all we wanted to do was be by their side and provide comfort.

I'd like to remind you of Joshua 1:9 *"The Lord your God is with you wherever you go."* You are not alone. Even though you may be sitting alone as you read this chapter, or perhaps there is a chance you are sitting alone in a hospital, you are not alone. Maybe you have a husband, wife, or child who is alone tonight and in pain. Although your heart wants more than anything to be next to their side, there may be physical constraints or barriers, and you cannot give the comfort you wish to give; I'd like to remind you that Joshua 1:9 is written for them as well. *"The Lord, your God, is with them wherever they go."* They are not alone; you are not alone. We trust and hope in the unseen One.

There is no such thing as a free lunch—or is there?

"On this mountain the Lord Almighty will prepare a feast of rich food for all peoples, a banquet of aged wine—the best of meats and the finest of wines."

Isaiah 25:6 NIV

Free food!!! We all love free food!!! Am I the only that believes that somehow the calories don't count when it's free? When we were moving early in our marriage, we convinced friends to come and help us by saying, "we'll buy you pizza and beer." That was enough for a full day of physical labor moving furniture. We've probably all heard of the saying, "There is no such thing as a free lunch," which rings true for most situations...*but maybe not always.*

Sal was in third grade doing online school during COVID-19 in the fall of 2020. He won an award at his school called "Top Pops," where his teacher provided recognition to him in front of the whole school during their chapel ceremony. It was an exceptional time. Also, one of the most coveted things about getting Top Pop is you get to each lunch with the other students who also got Top Pop and sit at a designated table with the Head of School. Wow! For third graders, this was their version of pizza and beer.

Since Sal was a digital learner, most of his classmates were back in the physical school, but he was still completing his classes by Zoom. On Sal's award day, we arranged with his teacher and the head of school that he could Zoom in for lunch and still get a chance to be included (even if via Zoom) and eat lunch with the head of school. Sal was so excited to participate. His teacher dismissed everyone for lunch, and then we got the Zoom all situated so he could be at the lunch table (via Zoom) and see the other "Top Pops" students and the head of school.

A couple of minutes before the official lunchtime, there was a knock at the door. I went down to open the door, and there was a delicious bag of food on our porch. It appeared someone had left a restaurant-style lunch for us. I brought the bag into the house. My mom, Sal, and

I opened it up, and it smelled so delicious and filled the house with flavor. It was perfectly cooked sparkling fried chicken with potato wedge fries that were heavenly and seasoned corn on the cob. There was enough food for the three of us. The mood in the house was so joyful, and my mom and I just assume this was for us. We thought the school had bought food for Sal for his special award, and sure enough, we got to partake in the delicious food as well. We all had our fill. We kept saying how good the food tasted and just somehow felt like we were deserving of this food that just showed up at the door. Sal was the only one living in reality and kept saying, "I don't think this is our food, mom." I responded, "Of course, it's our food, it was left at our door."

After about 20 minutes, I heard another knock on the door after all the food was gobbled up. I opened the door and there was a fence repairman who was hired by our Homeowners Association to fix the fences in our neighborhood. He looked exhausted and sweaty as he had been working all morning. He politely asked, "Ma'am, did you happen to see some food that was dropped off here at your doorstep?" My heart sank... we had just eaten his lunch. Oh My Gosh! I quickly confessed and profusely apologized. I said, "I am so sorry; we thought it was for us. We ate it, and it was delicious." I offered to order him another lunch, but the place delivery time had passed. We brought him water, chips, and fruit to give him something to eat and he just very professionally said, "That's ok, thanks." He was working near our house, so he used our address to have his food delivered. I felt so embarrassed. Then I was even more embarrassed about my attitude; somehow, I thought we deserved that lunch. Have you ever had a situation like this? Who are you in this story? Are you the worker who got cheated out of his lunch? Maybe you feel you got cheated out of something in life? Perhaps you feel cheated that your family has to face cancer and no one else does; why us? Or maybe you are Sal in the story. You know this isn't yours, and you do not deserve it. You are the voice of truth saying, "Something isn't quite right." Or, maybe, you are my mom and me. We just ate someone else's lunch full-throttle – something is seriously wrong with us. Guilt is now setting in, but somehow at the moment, it felt like the right thing to do. Who do you relate to most in the story today? What are you facing today?

I think about the words of Jesus and the banquet that awaits. In Isaiah, we are given a glimpse of the feast that is to come. Isaiah 25:6 says, *"On this mountain the Lord Almighty will prepare a feast of rich food for all peoples, a banquet of aged wine—the best of meats and the finest of wines."* Salvation awaits us, and I can't help but notice; isn't it funny that even in heaven, God promises us free

There will be no cancer, no tears, no pain, and no hospitals in heaven.

food – we get free lunch, although there was a cost paid for by the cross of Jesus Christ. There will be no cancer, no tears, no pain, and no hospitals in heaven. The feast is going to be better than anything we have ever tasted. The grace of Jesus is the sweetest victory for us all.

Practical Tip – Source of Comfort and Resources

Only 4% of Cancer Research goes to Childhood Cancer. We need more than 4%! Below is a list of non-profit organizations to help your family as you face childhood cancer. These organizations invest in things such as research, resources, experiences, and daily needs for your family. Please check out the unabridged resources in the appendix of this book for additional support as you take one step at a time.

- Evan Avenger's
- Wipe Out Kid's Cancer
- Hope Kids
- Social Worker in the hospital
- Stephen's Ministry at our local church

Notes

1   "Acute Lymphoblastic Leukemia: Chemotherapy Phases," *About Kids Health*, updated on March 6, 2018, https://www.aboutkidshealth.ca/article?contentid=2846&language=english#/.

2   "Pancreatic Cancer is a Silent Killer – and Other Myths," *Pancreatic Acton Network*, updated April 10, 2018, https://pancreaticcanceraction.org/news/myths-about-pancreatic-cancer/.

3   "Survival Rates for Pancreatic Neuroendocrine Tumor," *American Cancer Society*, updated January 26, 2021, https://amp.cancer.org/cancer/pancreatic-neuroendocrine-tumor/detection-diagnosis-staging/survival-rates.html.

Chapter 5

Resiliency: To Endure the Insurmountable

…I am the voice of perseverance.

I am here. Helping you rise again and again. Keep going, don't stop; I am steady and focused. I am not easily distracted. Reminding you to stay the course, I am here to help you. What you are facing today is manageable. You will persevere! No storm lasts forever; follow the way. The victory will be so sweet in the end.

Keep Moving Forward: Even if it Feels Like Going Backward

"When Mary came where Jesus was and saw him, she knelt at his feet and said to him, "Lord, if you had been here, my brother would not have died." When Jesus saw her weeping, and the Jews who came with her also weeping, he was greatly disturbed in spirit and deeply moved. He said, "Where have you laid him?" They said to him, "Lord, come and see." Jesus began to weep.

John 11: 32–35 NRSV

"Lord, if you had been here…if only you had been here, this would not have happened!" I have heard myself saying these exact words but with different details. "Lord, if only you had prevented cancer. If only you had protected Sal. Lord, if only you had saved my dad. Lord, if only you had been there with Alex…Lord, if only…if only; there were a million other ways I saw this playing out. If only you had shown up on my timing! How did I end up here?" The question circles in my head over and over. Have you ever been there? Perhaps you are facing an obstacle that looks like a step in the wrong direction. Scripture gives us insight into the depth of the human heart and a loving God who weeps with us during our sorrow. However, He still has a few things up His sleeve, ready to amaze us.

As we read the story further with Mary and Martha, we sense resentment and disappointment. Jesus let them down. You can sense the closeness between Jesus and Mary; there is a deep trust and brutal honesty. Mary knows Jesus had the power to heal her brother Lazarus when he was sick, and if only Jesus

Jesus' heart breaks when our hearts break.

had come sooner. From Mary's perspective, Jesus was late. He missed His chance. She needed Him there, and He didn't show up…although we know further into the story, *Jesus was right on time to display the work of God.* Jesus shows deep compassion for her and weeps with her. He knew he was not to blame for Lazarus' death. Jesus knew the power of God was about to wow them all. Yet, He still doesn't minimize her pain and hurt. Jesus' heart breaks when our hearts break. He weeps with Mary, and He weeps with us in our moments of bitter grief. We are not alone.

Lazarus' death was a gut-wrenching setback for both Mary and Martha; no rational person would describe this as progress. Yet, isn't it funny how "progress" is one of the most misleading words? We are conditioned that progress always means moving upward. It represents moving ahead. Progress is always moving forward, right? Not exactly. As with the story of Mary and Martha and in my own story, progress can sometimes feel like we are going backward. Progress is not always linear. This was not Mary and Martha's plan when their brother, Lazarus, died.. His death felt like going in reverse. How could the Lord not have come sooner? If only He had been there. Or maybe, just maybe, the Lord's timing was progress in disguise.

I remember a time with Sal when it felt that treatment was moving backward, not forward. We were in the ER as Sal had significant stomach pain and a fever. This was a different ER than we usually went to, so I was distrusting immediately. I went into the ER without positive intent. I was convinced those around us seemed uncaring. I was thinking, "Lord, how did we end up here? I don't want to be here!" I was in denial and just wanted to get the green light that everything was fine. Nothing to worry about. Stomach pain is expected on chemo, and we'd be released from the ER to go home that evening with some additional pain medication for Sal...*little did I know what was ahead.*

Sal's pain worsened, so they continued to give stronger pain medication. I sensed the nurse and doctor were frustrated with me as I was likely a pushy parent. But, the feeling was entirely mutual on my end, too, with them. They didn't seem to have the answer. My heart kept crying out to the Lord, "If only you had kept him healthy, if only we decided to go to the other ER. If only Lord...you had been here." After eight hours in the ER and an emotional roller coaster, the assisting doctor comes and says, "We're getting ready to discharge you. We can't determine the cause of pain, and it is likely just GI issues from chemo." I was thinking to myself. "It's about time. Let's get out of here. Yay! We're going home." My definition of progress at that very moment was going home.

But, before we got our discharge papers and as I was packing up the bag, the Head Doctor of the ER came into the room and said, "I am sorry, but something isn't right; I am overriding the decision. I am going to admit you into the hospital. I believe the stomach pain is hiding another infection, and we won't know until the labs are back. So, looks like you'll be staying here tonight or maybe a few more nights." What a setback! Seriously, we've been here for eight hours, and now you are sending us to be admitted! This felt like anything but progress.

> **What felt like a setback was protection in disguise.**

As it turns out, Sal did have a severe infection. He remained hospitalized for several more weeks on many antibiotics. God was there that night with us in the ER. God was there that night as the Head Doctor of the ER overrode the decision. What felt like a setback was protection in disguise. Below is an excerpt from my journal.

Journal Entry July 14, 2018

The ER was a disaster. I had to fight for him and be an advocate for him while it felt like no one was listening. Although someone was listening as God has put us where we need to be. We finally got up to our room at 2:30 am. Sal had a really hard day on Friday, and it was confirmed he has stomach issues, but more dangerously, he has a bacterial blood infection. We are in the hospital on the 6th floor, exactly where he needs to be. Regardless of the disaster it took to get up here, we are here, we are safe, and he is sleeping soundly. We have hope that tomorrow is a new day.

Progress rarely looked how we wanted it to look throughout the cancer journey. But wait, we can't stop reading the story of Mary and Martha…the twist is about to come! Jesus was right on time, and all those around, including Mary and Martha, witnessed a miracle…*progress towards healing and the Kingdom of God!*

"And Jesus looked upward and said, "Father, I thank you for having heard me. I knew that you always hear me, but I have said this for the sake of the crowd standing here, so that they may believe that you sent me." When he had said this, he cried with a loud voice, "Lazarus, come out!" The dead man came out, his hands and feet bound with strips of cloth, and his face wrapped in a cloth. Jesus said to them, "Unbind him, and let him go."

John 11: 41 – 44 NRSV

Progress in disguise, right? Do you see it? God's power was revealed through Lazarus' death. *Jesus was right on time.* Sal was in the hospital with a severe blood infection. This was the safest place for him to be. Jesus was not late to the party but showed us God orchestrated every step. God is weeping with you when you weep. God orchestrates the path forward in His timing, even if it feels delayed. And maybe, just maybe, setbacks are progress in disguise. We trust and hope in the victory that is to come.

Fear: Sometimes God lets the Storm Rage, and He Calms His Child

"The Lord is my light and my salvation; whom shall I fear? The Lord is the stronghold of my life; of whom shall I be afraid?"

Psalm 27:1 NIV

I have always been drawn to the scriptures that acknowledge fear because it is the human heart. It is the first emotion I felt when I heard the words, "Your child has cancer" or "Your husband has cancer." It's the first thing in the pit of your stomach when life is about to change. Even as we neared the end of treatment for Sal, I felt fear. What will the after-cancer experience feel like? What will it be like when the chemo isn't actively keeping cancer away? It's not surprising that "Do not fear" is also the first thing the angel says to Jesus' mother, Mary, when the messenger is about to tell her she will conceive through the Holy Spirit. The first words the angel says to the women at the empty tomb is "Do not fear, he is not here. He has risen!" I don't think it's an accident that the people in the Bible needed to hear the words "Do not fear," and it's no accident that we, too, need to hear the words "Do not Fear" often. Throughout both Sal and Alex's journey and even after the cancer experience, I still need to be reminded not to fear daily. It reminds me of one of my favorite bible stories of Jesus and his disciples.

Jesus Calms the Storm (Mark 4:35 – 41) NLT

As evening came, Jesus said to his disciples, "Let's cross to the other side of the lake." So they took Jesus in the boat and started out, leaving the crowds behind (although other boats followed). But soon a fierce storm came up. High waves were breaking into the boat, and it began to fill with water.

Jesus was sleeping at the back of the boat with his head on a cushion. The disciples woke him up, shouting, "Teacher, don't you care that we're going to drown?"

When Jesus woke up, he rebuked the wind and said to the waves, "Silence! Be still!" Suddenly the wind stopped, and there was a great calm. Then he asked them, "Why are you afraid? Do you still have no faith?"

The disciples were absolutely terrified. "Who is this man?" they asked each other. "Even the wind and waves obey him!"

This story has different layers to unravel. The first thing I like to point out is that scripture clarifies that Jesus is not just resting; He is in a deep sleep on a cushion. (I like the part about the cushion – it gives another added punch that Jesus is comfortable). The disciple's moment of complete fear when the storm is the loudest shows the dichotomy of Jesus sleeping on a cushion. I completely relate to the disciples at this moment in the story. The storm was hitting hard on this journey, and I looked around to the One who could save; where was Jesus? Jesus was asleep on a cushion. Does it ever feel like God is sleeping on the job? The disciples are preparing to die in the storm, so they wake Jesus and say, *"Don't you care if we drown?"* I remember yelling out to God, "Don't you care anymore! Don't you care? I see the pain in my husband's eyes. I see the suffering my son has endured. Don't you see what is going on…can't you do something? Don't you care if we drown!"

Jesus wakes up, and he doesn't reprimand the disciples…If He did, I wonder if it would go something like this, "Bros, come on, seriously, you woke me up for this? Leave me alone; I'm tired." No, Jesus immediately addresses their fear in just three words "Quiet, Be Still."

Even in the original Greek language, it is three words "ησυχία μείνε ακίνητος."

Note the next part of the scripture. The disciples were utterly terrified, *"Even the wind and waves obey him."* The disciples start out afraid and call on Jesus (who is sleeping on a cushion), and then Jesus calms their fear but now…they are even more terrified after witnessing the miracle. The extraordinary power of God at work. When we experience the supernatural, those unexplainable things that happen in our lives sometimes leave us even more awestruck and shocked. Below is an excerpt from my journal on my fear.

March 13, 2020

I write this from Alex's hospital room. I have wrestled with fear many times in the past 18 months as we've gotten a lot of opportunities to spend time in many hospital rooms. In some ways, they are all the same yet different. Dallas Children's Hospital Oncology floor is filled with hope on the walls and pictures of superheroes and bright colors. The adult oncology floor, where we are currently with Alex, is much darker and a sense of sadness and despair as we have seen some of the difficult end-of-life news people are enduring. And lastly, a year ago we were in the ICU with my dad. It was filled was slow movements, quietness, and the shadowed face of mortality. Yet, in each of these fearful places, God is still working and God is present and reminds us victory is coming. There is HOPE ahead!

There is a popular quote from a Pastor who is a close friend of our family. In one of his sermons, Pastor Austin Kraft stated, "Sometimes God calms the storm. Sometimes He lets the storm rage, and He calms His child." If you have a storm raging right now and it feels like God is sleeping on a cushion, remember God is still in control; He is in the boat with you. Cast your cares on him and remember Psalm 27:1 (KJV), *"The Lord is my light and my salvation; whom shall I fear? The Lord is the stronghold of my life; of whom shall I be afraid?"*

———

I still struggle with fear and anxiety. I worry that relapse will occur or that another illness will happen. During treatment, I was full of fear that the chemo wouldn't work and this battle would end in a heavenly healing and not an earthly one. I had to be intentional to work through my fears. One of the neuroscientists I have studied about the brain and the biological response to fear is Dr. David

Rock. He does a lot of research and neuro-based science on the brain's response to change. He has partnered with the Neuro Leadership Institute and written several books about the brain's response to changing environments and leadership.[1] Dr. Rock discusses when we feel pain, fear, or if a significant change occurs, there is a physical-biological reaction to fear and an emotional reaction. This is intentional for our survival. The adrenaline rush prepares us for flight or fight when in a dire situation. He gives tips on managing stress highlighting his acronym, SCARF (Status, Certainty, Autonomy, Relatedness, and Fairness).[2] I applied some of his concepts throughout the cancer journey, and I felt all 5 cylinders of SCARF firing within me simultaneously. This triggered not only emotional stress but a biological response as well. The heart, brain, and biology are all connected. As a mom with a child with cancer, there is more than daily comforts that are sacrificed. I remember thinking through all the things that give me security in life and realizing it felt out of control.

Thinking through the SCARF acronym, let's start with the first one. My "status" was no longer secure. The things I was known for before cancer will need to go on hold, at least for a little while. The "certainty" of things

I had ownership of are now threatened. The "certainty" of keeping my job and "certainty" of our lifestyle was at risk. The "A" stands for "autonomy." Now it felt that there was no freedom to do anything except follow protocol and understand the complete constraints of childhood cancer. "R" is for "relatedness.' The circle of friends will change and grow smaller. My time and hobbies would need to pause, which also meant socially connecting with others. And lastly, "fairness"…nothing about this seems fair. Have you ever felt one or more of the SCARF cylinders firing inside?

Here is how I managed through it. I reached out to people who God had given me as support pillars. Those who would listen and help carry my burden. Other times, I would sit in silence in the hospital and tell myself, "Today, I am just going to simply be there for my son." It didn't require me to have a status or be certain of the future. It didn't require a level of autonomy or fairness. God's light and a reminder of hope and salvation show through even in those moments. The flicker of hope slowly calmed the fears.

I remember one week when we were preparing for a difficult time during Sal's treatment called Delayed Intensification. God still provided small comforts along the way when my fear was getting the best of me. The doctors and nurses prepared us for the worst. He likely would be hospitalized, and although we thought we had already overcome much of it, the worst was still ahead. In my head, I knew I should calm down. I kept telling my head, *"The Lord is my light and my salvation; whom shall I fear? The Lord is the stronghold of my life; of whom shall I be afraid?" Psalm 27:1.* But my heart wasn't hearing it. My heart was on autopilot, "Mayday, Mayday! Fear, panic – flight or fight." This was survival, and I couldn't switch it off.

One evening I remember Alex was working late, so it was just Sal and I eating dinner together at our square dining room table. Alex was usually our chef in our household, so when he had to work late, dinner was not always the best. However, I think this particular night, I made a superb box of Kraft Mac n Cheese (no judgment, please). I was a bit subdued and quiet; Sal was too. We were sitting together in comfortable silence. Sal finally spoke and told me something so profound yet so simple and genuine.

He said, "Mom, when someone goes to heaven, and they have cancer, I think God touches them and it goes away right away. For me, I think God still touches me, but it's going to take a little longer." Wow! Such wisdom, confidence in the Lord's healing, and encouragement for me. Healing was going to take time. It's just going to take a little longer...and so we wait...and while we wait... we will trust in the Lord.

Even when my eyes could not see, even when my ears could not hear, even when my head could not remember, and even when my heart was full of fear...God was saying, "Lisa, my child, do not fear. I am with you." If the words "Do not fear" are in the Bible multiple times (it is said at least 365 times), then before we go to bed each night, may we remember, *do not fear, God is with you.* He calms the storm, He calms his child, and He calms our fears...now close your eyes; it's your turn to be asleep on a cushion.

Mommy Guilt

"The steadfast love of the Lord never ceases, his mercies never come to an end; they are new every morning; great is your faithfulness"

Lamentations 3:22-23 NRSV

God's mercies are new every morning. The guilt and shame of yesterday do not need to follow us into the next day; Amen! Every day is a fresh start. I needed to hear these words time and time again. There is guilt that we carry around us, and we don't have to because the steadfast love of the Lord never ceases! This verse in Lamentation describes a time of destruction. The city of Jerusalem is in ruin. The author of Lamentations, likely the prophet Jeremiah, paints a cruel and pitiful time in the world when the people of God would not listen and there were injustices. Yet, Jeremiah continued to dare to HOPE and hold onto God's promises. In times of pain, suffering, cruelty, and shame, the author of Lamentations points us to the steadfast love of the Lord.

If you are a parent, you know that along with all the love and joy of parenting, there is also guilt and self-doubt along with reflective questions...*am I doing this right? How will I know until it's too late?* If you are like me, there are moments throughout my motherhood where I carried the burden of mommy guilt, and I want you to know that, you don't have to, and neither did I. *God's mercies are new every morning.*

When Sal was about 4 years old, we got him a Beta fish. It was his first pet, and he was so excited! Sal helped feed the fish, and he talked to it. He named the fish Roger, and then the nickname Rogey (pronounced Rah-gee) soon developed. I have no idea how the name, Rogey, came to be, but somehow that was the name. Rogey was a beautiful blue beta fish with dark and light shades of blue. He was the kind of fish that looked like he needed a haircut. Sal loved Rogey, and they quickly became friends.

One day, I cleaned Rogey's tank and had a disastrous mommy fail. The tank was thoroughly cleaned and I had fresh water in the tank, meaning I was about done. I was now ready for one of the final steps: putting the fish back into the newly cleaned tank. I got the net, but Rogey was a bit squirmy that day. Before I could do anything about it, I don't know how it happened, but I dropped Rogey. He squirmed out of the net and landed on the counter. I am pretty sure Rogey bounced several times in my moment of utter panic. Alex was there watching the whole thing with his jaw on the floor. I quickly grabbed this slippery fish and got him back into the tank. My brain told me, "Quick, get the tank back in his room." I was just rushing to put this whole experience behind me. In my moment of haste, I forgot to add the critical water conditioner to make the water safe for the fish – a decision I will regret soon. I quickly put Rogey back onto Sal's dresser in his room as if nothing had happened. Yay! Rogey is all good, phew…*or so I thought.*

The next morning, Sal comes into our room, "Rogey is acting so weird. He is laying on the bottom of his tank and won't move." Oh no, I think. Alex and I go and check it out; sure enough, Rogey has died. We both know it before a word is spoken between us. But now, we must think through how we will explain this to a 4-year-old. What were we going to do with the fish – Yuck! We shared with Sal the basics of death, and there were tears and sadness. We kept it relatively simple but still had lots of empathy for a 4-year-old. Alex took care of the dead fish and we promised to get Sal another fish soon (just a little side note—we still haven't gotten a new fish; I think this experience was traumatic enough.) Later that day, when Alex and I were alone, he teasingly reminded me…I saw you drop Rogey. "What? No, I didn't," I said. I denied it immediately but then self-reflection set in. Oh My Gosh – not only did I drop the fish, but I also forgot the water conditioner. Oh no…I did it. I'm the one. I killed Rogey! I made a mistake. Have you ever made a mommy mistake that had a long-term consequence?

Here is how I managed it. The mommy guilt set in full-blown. I told Alex, "We will never share this with Sal and never speak of this again." I was embracing complete denial; let's pretend this never happened...what fish? Who's Rogey? Denial was my friend.

I carried that guilt with me for years! But, let me share the good news, I didn't have to! Some of you who are carrying guilt from decades ago or maybe even longer. So let me tell you, if you are having one of those days with a healthy dose of mommy guilt, let me just say, whatever you did or didn't do, just remember Rogey, the poor fish. Give yourself some grace –God's mercies are new every morning! Nothing could be as bad as killing your child's first pet.

Give yourself some grace – God's mercies are new every morning!

When Sal was a bit older and going through chemo, and then through my dad's death, we chose to be candid with Sal about death and the joy of heaven that is to come. His only reference to death was what happened with Rogey. A little while later, Sal's endless questions and curiosity eventually tied back to his fish and then, of course, my dad. "Mom, why did Rogey have to die? Why did Bomps (the name he called my dad) have to die? Why is there death?" A question we were all thinking. I confessed about Rogey. I told him that I was probably the one that inadvertently killed Rogey. He said, "It is ok, mom." Sal displayed grace towards me. He then quickly negotiated for his next pet, "But, now can I have a dog because you killed my fish." Ha! Nice try, bud.

Even in our shame and guilt, we tend to carry it over into the next day.. May the verse in Lamentations remind us that we no longer have to carry the burden. Jesus has paid the price. *"The steadfast love of the Lord never ceases, his mercies never come to an end; they are new every morning; great is your faithfulness."* Lamentations 3:22-23 NRSV Whatever happened yesterday or the day before, there is mercy for you each morning. You do not need to beat yourself up or carry the mommy guilt anymore. You are set free, and salvation is coming.

Maybe it's not your guilt that has you in a mind loop preventing you from moving forward, but the grief of an unresolved death that has stopped you and you can't progress. I have asked God the same question about my dad. "Why God? Why did my dad have to die so soon? Why did you take him to heaven just when I needed him here? Lord, I needed my dad to be here for my son!" I have learned that God has an unknown side, and only He knows our days.

As the Psalmist writes in one of my favorite *Psalms 139: 15-16*, *"My frame was not hidden from you when I was made in the secret place, when I was woven together in the depths of the earth. Your eyes saw my unformed body; all the days ordained for me were written in your book."*

Our days are numbered, and the sting of death always feels too short. We have heaven waiting for us, and we carry those in our hearts who have gone ahead before us. We look forward to the day when we will be reunited again, and one day, those who have gone before us will usher us into heaven and say, "Come and let me introduce you to the one we know as Jesus – His steadfast love for you is never ceasing."

Learning to Lament

"I cried out to God for help; I cried out to God to hear me. When I was in distress, I sought the Lord; at night I stretched out untiring hands, and I would not be comforted… You are the God who performs miracles; you display your power among the peoples."

Psalms 77: 1-2, 14 NIV

If you pick up the Bible and flip right in the middle, you will likely open it up to Psalms. The Book of Psalms has the reputation of being the praise and joyful part of scripture (which it is much of the time). However, did you know that out of the 150 total Psalms, there are 42 that are prayers of Lament?[3] If you flip to any random chapter in Psalms, you will land on a lament approximately 30% of the time. This is statistically significant. What other things would you like to have a 30% chance of happening? How about a 30% chance of becoming a millionaire (actual statistic is somewhere between 6%–22% according to the Federal Reserve Board survey of consumer finance)?[4] How about a 30% chance of having twins (the actual statistics is less than 1%)?[5] How about a 30% chance of keeping your New Year's resolution (the actual statistics are again, much lower, about 8%).[6] Yes, these are all aspects of life we talk about or prepare for, yet they have less than a 30% chance of happening. If God has shown us that 30% of the Psalms are prayers of laments, then clearly, God is for hearing our lamentations. We should not be afraid or reserved from learning to lament. He is not offended or off-put by our raw, untamed, or blunt expressions. You may even see in scripture that God is *in favor of* laments as he dedicated even a whole book with the root word called Lamentations.

So, what is lamenting exactly? Lamenting is a passionate expression of grief or sorrow. It does not hide from the pain and inevitably looks toward the future in hope. Below are several of my go-to laments in scripture when I was at my darkest moments in both Alex and Sal's journeys. I hope they provide you an avenue to express your sorrow to the One who hears your heart.

Psalm 10 1 "Why, Lord, do you stand far off? Why do you hide yourself in times of trouble?"

Psalm 13: 1-2 "How long, Lord? Will you forget me forever? How long will you hide your face from me? How long must I wrestle with my thoughts and day after day have sorrow in my heart? How long will my enemy triumph over me?"

Psalm 70: 1 & 5 "Hasten, O God, to save me; come quickly, Lord, to help me…But as for me, I am poor and needy; come quickly to me, O God. You are my help and my deliverer; Lord, do not delay."

Psalm 71: 11, 12 & 14 "They say, "God has forsaken him; pursue him and seize him. Do not be far from me, my God; come quickly, God to help me…As for me, I will always have hope; I will praise you more and more."

During one of the pivotal points for both Alex & Sal, I learned more about myself through lamenting to God. This was in the spring of 2020. Alex was in the hospital for over a week, and we could not see him. He was fighting a severe infection. He finally started healing, and I was able to pick him up. Oh, the joy! I couldn't wait. It was so different without him…my heart missed my husband.

Other things were going on externally; I felt the world was out of control. COVID-19 was in full ramp up with no vaccine; my husband and son were at significant risk. My sister had already gotten COVID-19. Because of the risk, we had to isolate ourselves from everyone, including my sister and her family. My employer was going through a merger, so there was a feeling that my career was in limbo. Although I received assurance from my manager not to worry, it was always an unsettling time at work.

Additionally, racial protests were going on in America that impacted some very dear family and friends; I wanted a different world for Sal. I was worn out and exhausted. Life felt heavy as it did for many of you too.

Alex was settling into being back home after spending over a week in the hospital. We were in a constant mode timing IV antibiotics, pain medication, and checking for fever. The IV antibiotics required a bit of teamwork from all of us. Alex needed to get his antibiotics through his PICC line every eight hours. However, critical timing and steps were required before and after administering the antibiotics. The medication was refrigerated most of the time, but it needed to sit at room temperature for one hour before going into his PICC line. So, one of us had to take the medication from the fridge and let it sit on the counter for at least one hour before. Then the IV would take about one and a half to two hours to administer. So, if you calculate doing this three times a day, there were only about five hours between the different doses, which went on for six weeks. During those weeks, there was never a restful night's sleep, and we had multiple alarms for Alex and Sal.

Within a few days of Alex returning from the hospital, Sal was playing inside on our footstool in the living room when suddenly I heard a loud crack followed by a scream.

He was holding his arm in pain. I knew it was broken by the sound it made. This was his 2nd broken arm (which happened to be the same arm he broke the first time). I was loading Sal into the car for a return trip to the hospital, which I had just come from a few days earlier with Alex. X-rays were taken, and it was confirmed that Sal had a broken wrist. On the plus side, he was able to get a cool camo cast that he was very proud of. Because of chemo, the bones heal slower, taking a solid eight weeks in a cast and another four weeks in a brace.

The following day after the broken wrist incident, Alex and I got up in the morning and opened our windows to look outside. Our living room has three large windows that look out to the driveway at the rear of the house that is connected to our backyard. The large cottonwood tree in our backyard fell and hit my car in the driveway during the night. "Are you kidding me?" I was thinking. Not only was I feeling that we were facing internal battles, this now felt like external forces were out to get us. After several calls to a tree service place and inspecting the damage to the car, the tree was finally chopped down and the car ended up being fine with some bumps and scratches. However, the saga continued. As a result of the tree hitting the house near the garage, it had propelled ants onto our roof. We didn't realize it at the time, but within a couple of weeks, there was an ant infestation in the upstairs bedroom. They had gotten into the roof and walls. More calls to specialists and more money going down the drain. Anger, loneliness, and confusion set in…what is happening? Why does it feel like the world is out to get us? Have you ever felt this way?

> **But, through my prayers of lament, I found my *hope and strength* again.**

I remember sitting at my desk just feeling hopeless and learning to pour out my sorrow. Did everything get immediately better? Were all my problems solved? No, we still had money going to things I would rather not spend money on, and my son and husband were still in the midst of the battle. But, through my prayers of lament, I found my *hope and strength* again. Below is a poem I wrote during that time of hardship.

June 20, 2020 – Poem of Lament

Even in the face of uncertainty, God can be trusted

Even in Childhood Cancer and the innocence of my son,
God can be trusted

Even in my darkest night of weeping and disappointment,
God can be trusted

Even in the unexpected death of my Dad and untamed
grief, God can be trusted

Even in shame, anger, and deep sorrow, God can be trusted

Even in the mortality of my husband and the shock and
despair of Pancreatic Cancer, God can be trusted

Even when God does not intervene, God can be trusted

Even when the suffering is lonely and God does not answer,
God can be trusted

Even when the character of what I know about God is not
visibly seen, God can be trusted

Even when the pain is so personal it feels cruel, God can
be trusted

Even in a new normal that feels like a bitter battle, God
can be trusted

Even in a pandemic and fear, God can be trusted

Even in racial injustice and tormented heartbreak, God
can be trusted

Even in our yearn for hope and desire for righteousness,
God can be trusted

Even though He sent His own son to suffer and die for me,
God can be trusted.

Jesus is coming! Yet I still dare to hope. Victory Ahead!

Practical Tip – Learning to Lament

God can be trusted in what you are facing today. As you reflect on the emotions that are pulling at your heart; whether that be guilt, shame, anger, confusion, grief, or sorrow, may you know you are not alone? I have been there too. Listed here are 10 Psalms and reflection questions to research if you are amid internal and external hardships:

Psalms 10, 13, 22, 25, 31, 44, 71, 77, 86, 142

1. What is the Psalmist's cry for help or complaint?

2. How is it the same or different from what you are facing?

3. What is the Psalmist asking for? What is it you are asking for?

4. Where is the statement of trust and hope in the Psalm?

5. What does it show about God's love?

Notes

1   "Books," Dr. David Rock, accessed January 28, 2022, https://davidrock.net/books/.

2   "Use the SCARF Model to Understand Our Individual Triggers," *Childcare Technical Assistance Network*, reviewed on January 28, 2022, https://childcareta.acf.hhs.gov/systemsbuilding/systems-guides/leadership/leading-ourselves/scarf-model.

3   "Language of Lament in Psalms," *Oxford Handbook Online*, updated July 2014, https://www.oxfordhandbooks.com/view/10.1093/oxfordhb/9780199783335.001.0001/oxfordhb-9780199783335-e-007.

4   "Your Overall Chances of Becoming a Millionaire by Race," *Financial Samurai*, updated January 4, 2022, https://www.financialsamurai.com/chances-becoming-millionaire-by-race-age-education/.

5   "Seeing Double: How to Increase Your Chances of Having Twins," *Healthline*, updated December 15, 2020, https://www.healthline.com/health/pregnancy/chances-of-having-twins.

6   "New Years Resolutions," *Fox 54*, Study done by University of Scranton, updated December 29,2019, https://www.rocketcitynow.com/amp/article/news/8-of-people-stick-to-their-new-years-resolutions-whats-yours/525-46821443-35a8-41b4-a32d-c5aab2a8ed43.

Chapter 6

The Flicker of Hope: Keep the Faith

...I am the voice of hope.

I am a flicker of light that can overcome the darkness. When faced with the impossible, I shine through. When facing the mountain, I can see the top. When facing fears, lies, and hopelessness...I am there redirecting you to never give up. Each small action is never wasted. I see you. I bring optimism and confidence that Victory is coming. You are not alone in your waiting. I am there too...waiting, praying, and hoping.

Run your race

"Therefore, since we are surrounded by such a great cloud of witnesses, let us throw off everything that hinders and the sin that so easily entangles. And let us run the race with perseverance the race marked out for us, fixing our eyes on Jesus. The author and perfector of our faith."

Hebrews 12:1-2 NIV

She is the phlebotomist at Dallas Children's hospital; she has a gift! We saw her often. She and Sal would always tease back and forth. She was loud, full of joy, and had a big personality, but even more, she had a special gift. Do you wonder what it is? She could draw blood with minimal pain. Her role was to physically stick needles into kids all day long. Not something that most people would sign up for. She knew who she was and the value she brought. She knew how to "prick quickly" so the screams and the tears would not start. She had a way about her. In most scenarios, this would be a dreaded part of the hospital appointments, but she knew how to reduce the pain and bring joy. She was full of confidence, and she didn't need to run anyone else's race. She was running her race, fixing her eyes on her

Jesus by helping those around her by easing the pain... and we were so very grateful for her.

He is the admin at the front desk and in charge of the appointments. He has a gift! We saw him often when we would check-in or out for appointments. Do you wonder what his gift is? He brought a calm presence and showed kindness in his eyes. Facing the anxiety before appointments, checking in, or rushing to get out of the hospital, he was always willing to go the extra mile. "Can I get you a parking pass? Does your child need throw-up bags?" He has a quiet voice and a peaceful way about him. He didn't need to run anyone else's race. He was running his race, fixing his eyes on Jesus by bringing peace and comfort to the patient's parents...and we were extremely grateful for him.

She is the cleaning and facilities person at Dallas Children's hospital; she has a gift! We saw her many days when Sal was hospitalized. She always came in with her mop, and so respectfully, she would ask first if she could clean the room. "Yes," would be my answer. She always had a bit of a hum while cleaning and seemed to have music in her heart. She was thorough with disinfectant and always smiled at us. She asked about our day and talked about the weather. She was good at getting our minds off the reason we were in the hospital. She didn't need to run anyone else's race. She was running her race, fixing her eyes on Jesus by getting rid of germs and bringing a smile...and we were very grateful for her.

Growing up, my dad was one of the primary witnesses who showed me how to run the race with perseverance. My dad was my role model from a young age. He had gifts. Do you want to know what his gifts were? He was a good listener and observer and shared his wisdom with me. He loved Jesus with his whole heart. He was not afraid to take risks and was good at planning...even if the stubborn German in him showed up occasionally. He held firm to his convictions, and he was my teacher for life. I often remember sitting at the large kitchen counter for hours as a child and even into young adulthood. He would cook, and we would talk. We moved a couple times, but each new house always had a large kitchen counter. Dad loved to cook and try new recipes. He shared his world with me during these special everyday moments between father and daughter. These times prepared me to go into the world ahead. It wasn't always the big moments or the birthday parties that I remember most. But it was the small things I remember about my dad. It was the everyday habits and little interactions. These moments were meaningful. He threw off all that untangled and ran his race, fixing his eyes on Jesus until his very last breath....I am so grateful for him.

Just like each of the individuals I described, run your race. It isn't always the big visible things that will make an impact. It is the small everyday interactions you have with your child through cancer; it is the times you sit on the couch and just hold their hand for hours. It's when you watched their favorite movie with them for the 50th time, and by now, you can quote the whole thing. It's the small moments before bed each night where you say "I love you" or rub their head as they sleep. These are the moments that matter the most.

The verse in Hebrews, *"Therefore, since we are surrounded by such a great cloud of witnesses, let us throw off everything that hinders and the sin that so easily entangles. And let us run the race with perseverance the race marked out for us, fixing our eyes on Jesus. The author and perfector of our faith."* ...is beautiful imagery. This passage reminds us to throw those things out that entangle us and focus on the race ahead. I picture a runner shedding those things that entangle them, so by the end, they are free with arms wide open and a huge smile taking in the victory. I reflected on those things that have entangled me throughout this journey. At times it's been worry or fear. I have felt ensnared by a feeling of being inadequate or self-doubt. There have been moments of despair and hopelessness. I wrestled with each of those thoughts, and they slowed me down and kept me from fixing my eyes on the almighty physician, Jesus Christ.

You, too, are uniquely created to run your race. We don't always get to choose the race we get to run. Sometimes life chooses for us. Actually, most of the time, life chooses for us. So remember, you have a gift. Reflect on what it is. What do you uniquely bring into other people's lives? Maybe you are a prayer warrior and bring strength. Maybe you are goofy and bring the humor. Or, perhaps you are smart and provide solutions. Whatever it is…you have a gift. You don't need to run anyone else's race…. just remember…your child facing cancer is so *very grateful* for you (even those teenagers who may never let on).

If your child hasn't told you, or perhaps, they can't tell you, I will say it for them. *You are appreciated.* Run your race that is marked out for you, and I will run my race too.

It's ok to grieve… "This isn't supposed to be happening?"

"Blessed are those who mourn, for they will be comforted."

Matthew 5:4 NIV

It's April 2020 on Easter Sunday! We were in the parking lot of Baylor, Scott, & White hospital in Plano, Texas. I step out onto this small grass area, looking up at the large hospital nine floors high. This is where Alex is…*he was supposed to be home by now.* I miss him deeply. It has been over a week since he hasn't been home. The hospital is a large rectangle from the outside with layers of windows. There are many signs in the parking lot pointing to different areas. I see a sign that has an arrow with big letters saying, "ER." There is an area for a helicopter flight for life, and you can also see the helipad. On the other side of the hospital, there is a large parking structure. On our side, where I am standing, there is uncovered parking and circular patches of grass that fill the surrounding areas of the hospital. You can tell the architect wanted some vegetation and large areas of grass and plants to show life.

I keep thinking to myself, "We should have been home all together eating Easter dinner." There is a disappointment in the air. I feel a sense of sadness. Then I feel bad for feeling the way I do, and now I feel guilty for having self-pity. Has that ever happened to you? You start to over-analyze your feelings. I started questioning my feelings, and then it was this weird cycle of telling myself, "I should be feeling a certain way." It's ok to have multiple emotions simultaneously, even if those emotions are contradictory. My expectations were unmet. Alex should have been home doing Easter baskets and eggs. He wasn't, and I felt a profound loss. We didn't know it then, but it would be another ten days before he could come home.

It's ok to have multiple emotions simultaneously, even if those emotions are contradictory.

I called my sister earlier in the week, and we decided we would go to the hospital where Alex was and wave to him from the parking lot, so he knew we were rooting for him. I wanted to provide him encouragement and support even if we still had the hospital walls between us. I wasn't quite sure how this was going to work out. Would he be able to see us? How will we know what room he is in? I thought, "Let's do it; nothing hurts to try." We knew we were on the right side of the hospital as I had been inside the hospital when Alex first had his surgery and knew the room numbers and where he would be. I remember we got to the area, and I started counting the tiny squares representing the row of windows for each floor. I start counting…1,2,3…all the way to the 7th floor, near the very top. That is where he should be, maybe, I can't tell. I felt this was going to be a needle in the haystack. I remember thinking, "Hmm, this looks impossible." All the windows and rows looked the same. My heart yearned to be by him; I was going to show him how much I loved him by cheering. I remember thinking this was the closest proximity we had been all week as COVID restrictions still would not allow visitors into the hospital.

He looked out his window, and we must have been quite a sight to see. My sister unexpectedly pulled out a large American flag waving it around. I saw it streaming across the small grassy area while thinking of the beautiful bold colors. The white was so pure for God the Fathers' holiness, the gallant red stripes for the blood of Jesus, and the blue stars for the baptism of the Holy Spirit.

My spirits began to lift. My mom somehow found a bright light pink umbrella in the car that she was waving around. It was really windy that day, so the American flag swayed in the wind, and the umbrella flipped up the other direction and was inverted. Oh well, my mom just waved that umbrella proudly. We had to stay socially distanced, so we were lined up with space between us. My nephew and Sal were running on the grass and jumping off small areas of rocks and hilly grass. All of us were waving our arms in the air and our voices were loud (not that anyone in the hospital could hear us).

I am on the phone with Alex as he is looking out his window, and suddenly he says, "I see you! I see you!" His voice is filled with joy, and he begins laughing... such a wonderful sound. "You can see us?" I ask. "Yes, you can't miss it! I see you all." I felt such a sense of relief...but wait, I couldn't see him, though. I couldn't tell which room he was in. I think to myself, "God, give me something. Can you just give us a little flicker, so we know he is there?" Do you ever feel this way? You are looking up, just waving your arms, saying, "God, show me something, a wink, an affirmation, show me hope. Just give me something!"

Suddenly, I have an idea. I ask Alex to make his way to the light switch and turn his room light on and off so we can see which room. I am sure this was not an easy task for him as he was hooked up to an IV. But after a couple of minutes, suddenly, there it is, way up on the hospital wall. I see a tiny light flickering...It's him, a light of hope! We are not alone! We start dancing and jumping outside, and I have tears in my eyes. We lifted our arms in prayer and prayed for him and all those in the hospital. Alex had strength and joy in his voice. This was indeed an

> **I see a tiny light flickering...**
> **It's him, a**
> **light of hope!**

uplifting experience. I sense hope is coming by just a tiny flicker of light. *"Blessed are those who mourn, for they shall be comforted."* Matthew 5:4

We drive home that night, and my spirit is uplifted. But I also can't help but wish...this isn't right. This isn't what it should be. Have you ever felt that way? It's ok to grieve what might have been or what should have been. It's ok to mourn and feel lost during the valleys of life... God promises, *"Blessed are those who mourn, for they shall be comforted."* Matthew 5:4 NIV

A funny thought popped in my head several weeks later. Imagine if you were another patient on another floor who is desperately lonely and hasn't been allowed to have visitors. Imagine if you are one of the nurses who had an emotionally draining day working double shifts or a doctor who can see the treatment isn't working for their dear patients. Imagine you are one of them, walking down the hallway, and you glance out the window and see us! I am sure it was quite a surprise to see a family of eight of various ages dancing and waving flags and umbrellas. I am sure it caused someone to do a double-take. Perhaps someone else in the hospital was mourning, and this brought them comfort. Maybe they thought we were cheering for them, giving them the strength to keep fighting. Or, maybe, just maybe, we were a tiny flicker of light that hope was coming.

So, next time you find yourself in the hospital, don't be afraid to look out the window and imagine the angels in heaven waving their mighty wings and flaming swords and God cheering you on and providing comfort in the most unexpected ways. It's still ok to feel joyful and let a smile sneak in while simultaneously thinking...*this isn't supposed to be happening.*

God is still doing miracles today!

"Now to him who is able to do immeasurably more than all we ask or imagine, according to his power that is at work within us, to Him be the glory in the church and in Christ Jesus throughout all generations, forever and ever! Amen."

Ephesians 3:20 NIV

Corrie Ten Boom was a holocaust survivor. She and her family were Christians who helped many Jewish people by hiding them in their home during WWII. They were eventually discovered, and Corrie Ten Boom and her sister were sent to Ravenstruck Concentration Camp. Her sister did not survive.[1] After her release, Corrie wrote the book, "The Hiding Place." One of my favorite quotes she wrote is, "Never be afraid to trust an unknown future to a known God."[2] The power of God is at work in each of us. Even though our futures are unknown, the Lord promises He will do immeasurably more than we ask or imagine through His power within us. God is still doing miracles today (even if

> **"Never be afraid to trust an unknown future to a known God."**

it takes slightly longer than expected). Through it all, I can confidently say God is good! We have a merciful, loving, and hope-filled God.

Sal's cancer journey was the biggest soul-gripping shock of my life. I have seen God answer prayers in different ways. I fell on my knees and prayed and prayed…and prayed, "Lord, spare my son; please don't take him from me!" I pleaded with the Lord. It took over three years of treatment, and God showed us in visible and invisible ways that He was holding Sal's hand through the pain and every step of the way…and God was holding our hands too.

God is glorified even in our pain. There were moments when Sal should have been hospitalized or in ICU, but he wasn't…he was protected. God can do more than we can ever imagine. I like to think that Sal had an army of angels surrounding him. God is still healing today, even in pain, *"Now to him who is able to do immeasurably more than all we ask or imagine, according to his power that is at work within us, to Him be the glory in the church and in Christ Jesus throughout all generations, forever and ever! Amen." Ephesians 3:20 NIV*

My dad's death was unexpected and then followed by deep grief. When he was in the ICU, we were just waiting…waiting for a miracle. I fell on my knees and prayed and prayed, … and prayed, "Lord, spare my dad. Please don't take him from me!" God mercifully took my dad home to heaven. My prayer request was not answered the way I would have liked. However, God is still healing today and sometimes it means heavenly healing. My dad had run his race and kept the faith. God provided loving ways for us to be comforted and cherished memories of my dad that I hold dear. God is able to do more than we can ever imagine, even in death, *"Now to him who is able to do immeasurably more than all we ask or imagine, according to his power that is at work within us, to him be the glory in the church and in Christ Jesus throughout all generations, forever and ever! Amen."* Ephesians 3:20 NIV

Alex's cancer journey felt cruel and lonely. I had my slew of doubts and candid conversations with God. I fell on my knees and prayed and prayed… and prayed, "Lord, spare my husband; please don't take him from me!" The Lord spared Alex. However, the suffering was long, and the healing took time. God is still with us through it all, and I know he never let us go. He gave us the strength to tackle each day and gave Alex the perseverance to keep holding on. God is still doing miracles today, even in suffering. *"Now to him who is able to do immeasurably more than all we ask or imagine, according to his power that is at work within us, to Him be the glory in the church and in Christ Jesus throughout all generations, forever ever and ever! Amen." Ephesians 3:20 NIV*

I don't know what the future holds for you and me. It may have more heartache, more suffering, and more pain. Perhaps it will have more joy, more stability, and more laughter. We had a running joke with our oncologist when we would see her for Sal's checkups. She would ask, "How was the weekend?" Sometimes we would answer, "Boring." She would smile and say, "Boring is good! We like boring here."

Interestingly, throughout this journey, I have come to appreciate boring too. I remember being so bored during the summers as a child with nothing to do until it would make me go stir crazy. I used to hate to be bored. To be honest, though, I am ok if perhaps there are a few dull days ahead for us. We've had plenty of adventure so far.

Who knows, regardless of what life unfolds, I have learned to surrender and take Corrie Ten Boom's words to heart… "Never be afraid to trust an unknown future to a known God." God has abundant plans ahead to give us hope and a future.

"Now to him who is able to do immeasurably more than all we ask or imagine, according to his power that is at work within us, to Him be the glory in the church and in Christ Jesus throughout all generations, forever and ever! Amen."

Ephesians 3:20 NIV

Team Grandma is on the Way

"He will wipe every tear from their eyes. There will be no more death or mourning or crying or pain, for the old order of things has passed away."

Revelation 21:4 NIV

It was Labor Day weekend in September 2020 and several things converged simultaneously. Sal was still on chemotherapy. Due to COVID-19, we chose to have him attend a new school, Prince of Peace Christian School in Carrolton, Texas as a digital learner for third grade. He had just begun the first few weeks of school as fully remote, and attending via Zoom was a difficult adjustment. I was working from home full-time, and like many other moms during this time, I was balancing

full-time work and trying my best to be a pseudo teacher
to my son. My office space was upstairs, so we chose to
have Sal across the hallway from me. This was purpose-
ful, so I could keep an eye on him and, most of all, hear
everything going on. His class was in-person. However,
Sal and sometimes other students were on Zoom. It was
a blended environment.

It's fascinating to suddenly be thrust into third grade
again as a fly on the wall. I got a glimpse into what Sal
was learning, but my favorite part was hearing the questions and commotion that would arise from the third
graders. Like the time a dragonfly somehow got into the
classroom. You would have thought it was a tornado by
the class's reaction with high-pitched screams and kids
jumping out of the way. But his teacher, Pam Knotts,
was so steady and calm, "third graders, it's only a dragonfly." Another entertaining event occurred when a few
kids learned to whistle and showed everyone else. Mrs.
Knotts, knowing third graders so well, reminded them,
"It's a wonderful thing to whistle, but you need to save
that for recess." Or the time their class pet, Hershey
the Guinea Pig, got to roll around in a ball across the

classroom floor. Hershey was well-loved and so much fun for third graders!

There was also some sadness and hard life lessons. One day, Mrs. Knott discovered that Hershey had died in his sleep during the night. It was a sad day for those third graders as many experienced grief for the first time and could openly share their emotions. Mrs. Knotts navigated it remarkably. I remember hearing it on Zoom, and I will admit, I even had a tear in my eye for these kiddos. However, it's a reminder that our sadness can still turn to joy. Shortly after, Mrs. Knotts brought a new Guinea Pig. The class got to be the first class to pick her name...Snowball won the most votes (another solid lesson in democracy and the popular voting system)... Snowball it is. Every day there was something adventurous that happened. I want to give a huge shout-out to all those teachers out there. I have learned that teaching elementary school is not my gift, and you are all truly a blessing from God. An extra special shout-out to Mrs. Pam Knotts. She was an answer to prayer and is not only a gifted teacher but has become as close as family to us.

When school started in August, my mom was in Colorado as she was spending part of her retirement there for several months. Alex was transitioning back to work, which was a trying time for us as a family. We were on our own; however, I really thought we were through the worst of it. Surely, from what we had been through, I thought I could handle whatever came next. What was lurking around the corner? Do you ever get the feeling that something bad is about to happen, but you just can't seem to shake it?

Also, due to COVID-19, we couldn't be indoors with my sister and her family. So, we scheduled some social distance outdoor visits with masks just so we could at least see another human being and satisfy my extraverted craving for social contact. Some of you probably had similar experiences. We had been quarantined for so long that I realized I began looking forward to my new version of girl's night out, which was the weekly drive to the pharmacy down the street with the music blasting in the car singing at the top of my lungs. I know I could have probably gotten the prescriptions delivered to the house; however, this was a glimpse of normalcy just to pick up the medications for Alex and Sal. Goodness, you know it's terrible when the pharmacy becomes your favorite hangout spot.

Alex was back at work full-time but was still not 100%. The doctors never did find the source of his infection, so it felt like we were living on borrowed time. What else could possibly go wrong? How much more pain and tears were left? I remember Alex came home from work before the Labor Day holiday, and it felt like we were going backward. He didn't look well; I could see it in his eyes. The other shoe was about to drop. He spiked a fever that night, so we again drove him to the ER. And yet again, I was not allowed to go in with him, and Sal and I watched from the car as he, once again, slowly walked inside. We knew the drill as this was not our first rodeo. I waited for a couple of hours with my cell phone glued to my hand for his text of the dreaded news. Sure enough, it came, and it was the update I feared. It read, "The CT scan showed more fluid. The infection is back. I am being admitted and don't know how long I'll be here. Will call later; Luv you, Babe."

… At that moment, I broke. I couldn't hold it together. I wept.

Who do you call in your moment of desperation? Who do you go to when the world crashes; who did I call? I called my mom; she listened. Shortly after, I immediately called my mother-in-law. My mom and mother-in-law were in Colorado, located about 20 minutes apart. Colorado is where Alex and I both grew up. I don't remember the exact words that were spoken, but the message I heard back from them was, "Hold on just a little longer; I am on the way!" I think my mother-in-law may have even said, "If I have to walk, run, take a train, or bus…I am coming." It was a tremendous relief for me; I knew help was on the way! I only had to just hold it together a little while, and soon help would be here. I told Sal the following morning, "Help is coming! Your Grandmas will be here soon…Team Grandma is on the way!"

> **"Hold on just a little longer; I am on the way!"**

I can only imagine the sight. My mom and mother-in-law are both petite in height but feisty in spirit. My mother-in-law has short brown hair and is about my height. My in-laws live on a farm with chickens, cows, and sheep that they care for while tending the land. My mother-in-law, Jackie, has a true gift of teaching and leads multiple bible studies. And, of course, I have to mention, she sure loves her red Prius. My mom, Kathy, is shorter than me (about 5 feet) with short gray hair. Our family jokes that my mom has the gift of "opinion." You never have to guess where my mom stands on any given topic; she'll share it with you generously. But seriously, all kidding aside, she truly has wisdom and a servant's heart that I admire and try to emulate. Both have a meaningful place in my life, and both moms were needed. Team Grandma loaded into that red Prius that day and took the 14-hour road trip from Colorado to Texas. I heard about a few incidents. There was a heavy rainstorm they had to pass and something about a windshield wiper incident where one flung off and needed to get repaired. That's just minor for the unyielding Team Grandma... nothing was going to hold them back.

Team Grandma was a tangible flicker of light that help was on the way. They were on the way to wipe my tears, they were on the way to be there in our pain, and they were there to make it better. I don't have to hold onto the old order anymore. They would be here to bring a new refreshing and illuminating hope. Their arrival reminded me of the verse above from Revelation. *"He will wipe every tear from their eyes. There will be no more death or mourning or crying or pain, for the old order of things has passed away." Revelation 21:4 NIV*

This scripture describes another team for us... *Team Trinity (Father, Son, and Holy Spirit).*

Team Trinity is on the way in our moment of desperation. Team Trinity has already prepared a place for us with lots of rooms, a place called heaven. There is no crying and no pain. A place where there are no hospitals because it's not necessary. There is no sickness. It's a place where there is no chemo because there is no cancer. There is no sorrow, grief, or sadness; there is only hope. Salvation is waiting for us. We have heaven coming, and Team Trinity has made a way through the unyielding abundant grace that only God can give through the resurrection of Jesus Christ. Hold on just a little longer... *help is on the way.*

Practical Tip:

Tips to Cope as a Family After-Cancer

We allowed Sal to try something new he had never done before. He signed up for basketball, and we were carefree. Sal met new friends, and we allowed him to share with them about Leukemia if he wanted to. Sometimes he shared openly; however, other times, he didn't share as that was no longer his primary identity. This was a shift for me too. I had been known as a "medical mom" for over three years. I was a caretaker; my identity was in my child's cancer. However, Sal no longer had cancer. What was I going to be known for now? For starters, Sal chose to be known as a great basketball player, and I guess I will have to shift too. I will be known as his proud mom (and, of course, I'm the mom who is cheering louder than any other parent in the stands).

Tips and Quotes from Others

"My daughter was so little when she got cancer, about 18 months old, that she doesn't remember any of it. I remember it clearly and she only knows what we tell her and show her pictures from the experience." (Dad of a daughter who had cancer).

"We took a family vacation to Disney World and went all out! This was our time to celebrate being together." (Mom of a daughter who had cancer)

"I started a non-profit organization for the child-hood cancer cause. This has become my passion and I want to keep helping others who are facing cancer." (Mom of a son who had cancer)

"My son was a teenager when he got cancer and did not want to share it with others and did not want us to share it broadly either. He barely told his best friend what he was going through and why he was no longer at school. I am choosing to respect his decision, so we have tried to adapt. He has 6 months of chemo and then we'll see." (Mom of a son who has cancer)

"If I had to have coffee with a friend who just found out their grandson had cancer I would tell them God will not let go of your child, grandchild, or you. His love is stronger and deeper than anything we can imagine. His plan is always in the best interest of our souls. I would listen and after coffee would go home and pray for them." (My mom, grandma of grandson who no longer has cancer)

Notes

1   "Corrie Ten Boom Biography," *The Biography*, accessed February 2, 2022, https://www.biography.com/activist/corrie-ten-boom.

2   Corrie Ten Boom Quotes. BrainyQuote.com, BrainyMedia Inc, 2022, accessed February 2, 2022, https://www.brainyquote.com/quotes/corrie_ten_boom_381184.

Chapter 7

Victory is Ahead: Dare to Hope

…I am the voice of Victory!

It is I, the peace that passes all understanding. It's the time of celebration and jubilee! Cancer has been crushed–the trauma, the pain, the insecurity, and loss of control–the greatest deception is defeated. I am the redemption in this world. Strength, perseverance, and hope brought us to this moment. There was never a time when you were alone. One day, all that is wrong in this world will be made right. I offer you Victory! I am Yahweh, Adonai, and Sovereign Lord. I was there at the beginning and am here now…the great "I am."

Do you see Sal's parents sitting there in the hospital – this same hospital where they sat over three years ago when their life changed? I am there too and today it's filled with smiles and joy. Sal will ring the bell! We will all be cheering as he now finished with treatment. The greatest deception is destroyed. Cancer is not welcome here today, there is no darkness.

I am the voice of Jesus. I will be with you always to the very end of the age.

Victory is Ahead!

There is a Superhero in us All

"For in hope we were saved. Now hope that is seen is not hope, because who hopes for what he sees? But if we hope for what we do not see, we eagerly wait for it with endurance."

Romans 8: 24-25 NET

When you hear the word *hope*, what do you think of? Do you think of joy, wishful thinking, a possible outcome, or is hope an anchor for you? The rock and truth that you hold onto! The scripture in Romans 8 is not another form of wishful thinking... *"For in hope we were saved."* It is not referring to an unknown outcome or uncertain term. We use the word, hope, sometimes too loosely, for example, "Hey, you gonna watch the cowboys' game today? I sure *hope* they win." That is not the kind of hope Paul shares in the book of Romans. He is speaking about the grit of hope, a *flicker* stronger than any darkness. This tenacious and illogical hope is both compelling and compassionate at the same time. This *hope* is our source of truth! We wait patiently, knowing we will dare to hope because it takes bravery to keep fighting, courage to move forward, and hope to be victorious.

We had a rule in our house that Sal could wear whatever he wanted to the hospital during his chemo and procedure days. During most of his treatment, he wore superhero costumes. We had Darth Vader, many different Star Wars characters, Mario, Superman, Capes, and all sorts of outer garments representing victory and hope. We had many different capes and masks that looked strong and intimidating. Some of the costumes had carved muscles and big shields. Sal was already a conqueror in our eyes, but this was a tangible way to show victory was coming because he was a walking super-hero. Sal would walk proudly at the hospital in his costume and make the nurses and doctors guess which super-hero he was that day. Some of them nailed it every time…they knew their super-hero list! Seeing Childhood Cancer firsthand and being part of the sub-culture of families also experiencing this path, there is no doubt…our children facing cancer are our super-heroes! (By the way, the other perk we learned about Superhero costumes is many of them have a head-cover or mask which covers up having no hair). I loved that Sal enjoyed the costumes. It gave a small glimpse of imagination and creativity. We had tons and tons of superhero costumes. This sparked joy for us as a family and a tiny flicker that *hope* was coming; victory is around the corner.

Then, one day, when Sal was in second grade and during a portion of treatment when he could partially attend school, he came home and said, "Mom! They are doing super-hero day at school, and we get to dress up." "That's great," I responded while thinking about which costume he would pick since we had many to choose from. He didn't have one favorite costume as it would vary by the week sometimes which one was his favorite. Sal confidently asked if he could dress up as his super-superhero. "Well, who was that?" I asked. Sal responded, "I would like my own pair of hospital scrubs because dad wears hospital scrubs, and all the hospital workers, nurses, and doctors that help me wear scrubs." "Wow," I thought and just paused. He knew who was rooting for him.

The support, particularly from one of our nurse practitioners, became an anchor for us. She always brought a balanced hope based on truth and reality, but Sal could always get her to laugh and smile. Her discernment and guidance are what we relied on time and time again. She was our superhero, and I know it was no mistake that we were paired up with her as one of her patients. Her impact will never be forgotten.

It's amazing how the hospital workers and nurses were looking to Sal as a super-hero fighting cancer, but all along, they were heroes to him in his life. Each of them mattered to us. They each were a tangible reminder of *hope*. They not only provided expertise and honesty when we needed to hear it but above all, they always viewed our journey through the eyes of victory. I knew they were rooting for us; I felt it…and so did Sal. Without delay, we got Sal a pair of navy-blue kid-size scrubs (Thank you, Amazon Prime)! That morning getting ready for school, Sal confidently put on his scrubs. He had his kid's sneakers on with the velcro strap. He loaded up his backpack and carried his lunch box by his side. Sal was ready to go and excited to be a superhero! He was the only child not in a cape that day at school and he proudly wore his hospital scrubs.

You may be someone reading this book, and you have lost your hope along the way. Maybe it's there, but it is a tiny, calm, steady flicker. It's not cliché; there is a superhero in us all. God uniquely made you for this race that you are in. God is here with us, and we are made in His image. God already won! He knows victory is ahead, so we can confidently hold onto a secure and unyielding *hope...* and try our absolute best to wait patiently for the victory to come. The scripture states, *"For in hope we were saved. Now hope that is seen is not hope, because who hopes for what he sees? But if we hope for what we do not see, we eagerly wait for it with endurance." Romans 8: 24-25 NET*

> **God uniquely made you for this race that you are in.**

So, throw a cape on today (or hospital scrubs), and we will DARE to HOPE with you.

All Clear

"What no eye has seen, what now ear has heard, and what no human mind has conceived -the things God has prepared for those who love him..."

1 Corinthians 2: 9 NIV

The doctor said All Clear! There was NED (No Evidence of Disease). The CT scan was all clear. Such beautiful words to the ear. I can just hear them over and over again. I never want to forget that moment. Praise God! Alex no longer had cancer. The oncologist did not mince his words and was straightforward and laid out a surveillance plan. We'll do scans every six months, and then we'll see. In other words, he was saying, "Go, live your life. Nothing is stopping you now." I remember we got in the car and drove home, and it felt joyous and happy, but also it was strange. I was so used to fighting cancer; what happens now? What happens when there is no cancer to fight? Is this what being cured feels like? Is this what we call healing? What does this now mean for us? Multiple questions began to arise in my head. Do we go back to life before cancer? Utterly impossible. We cannot possibly know what God has prepared for us, but as scripture says, *"What no eye has seen, what no ear has heard, and what no human mind has conceived -the things God has prepared for those who love him..." 1 Corinthians 2: 9 NIV*

In the Old Testament, there is a story of King Hezekiah in 2 Kings, Chapter 20. King Hezekiah had a boil and was ill and sick. The prophet Isaiah comes to him and informs him he will die, and he will not recover. Hezekiah prays to the Lord, and through Isaiah, the Lord says, *"I will heal you. On the third day from now you will go up onto the temple of the Lord. I will add fifteen years to your life."* *2 Kings 20: 5-6 NIV* God heard his request and listened. Then Isaiah prepares a poultice of figs, which are applied to the boil, and King Hezekiah recovers. In other words, King Hezekiah was All Clear! He had NED (No Evidence of Disease)! This was God's miraculous healing through the figs...a single dose of medicine. A reminder that no eye has seen, no ear has heard, and no mind can imagine how God chooses to heal. These must have been the most beautiful words to King Hezekiah. I wonder if King Hezekiah thought, "What does life look like now? Is this healing?" It is all counted as progress. Scripture gives some additional insight into what the next 15 years held for Hezekiah, and it does not show peace and security in his lifetime. However, there are still accomplishments noted, and King Hezekiah ultimately rests with his ancestors. God heals, and sometimes it takes just a single dose.

In the New Testament, there is a story about a blind man that Jesus heals. *"They came to Bethsaida, and some people brought a blind man and begged Jesus to touch him."* *Mark 8: 22 NIV* (God heard their request and listened).

"He took the blind man by the hand and led him outside the village. When he had spit on the man's eye and put his hands on him, Jesus asked, "Do you see anything?" He looked up and said, "I see people; they look like trees walking around." Once more Jesus put his hands on the man's eyes. Then his eyes were opened, and his sight restored, and he saw everything clearly." Mark 8:23 – 25 NIV The blind man was All Clear! He had No Evidence of Disease! This was God's miraculous healing…even if sometimes a second dose is required. These must have been wonderful words to those who saw this miracle firsthand. I wonder if the blind man thought, "What does life look like now? Is this healing?"

Scripture does not detail what happens to the blind man, but I can only envision he didn't go back begging in the street. He was changed! He was All Clear. I wonder if the formerly blind man became an artist because he can now see color, or maybe he became an architect because he can see shapes. Or, perhaps he went home and loved his family wholeheartedly and was grateful every day to the Lord Jesus because he could now see and touch his loved ones' precious faces. Who knows what progress was for him, yet still a reminder that no one can imagine how

God chooses to heal, and in this situation, he needed a second dose. *"What no eye has seen, what now ear has heard, and what no human mind has conceived -the things God has prepared for those who love him..."* 1 Corinthians 2: 9 NIV

In 2021, my precious son Sal finished his chemotherapy! He was 9½ years old. He had over three years of active chemotherapy (1165 days, to be exact). This included over 1000 doses of oral chemo and over 35 chemo infusions through his port. He had 22 lumbar puncture procedures, ten ER visits, and three ambulance rides. He had two surgeries and two bone marrow biopsies. He spent 39 nights hospitalized, had six blood transfusions, and had one hair loss episode. As a family, we had countless sleepless nights. Yet, God still provided an abundance of hope. Sal is a Leukemia survivor. Sal is All Clear! The greatest deception, Childhood Cancer, was defeated...the greatest fall from victory. The flicker of hope claimed victory. Sal is now in remission and off treatment. No more chemo. Hallelujah! This was God's miraculous healing...even if sometimes it took multiple doses over three years.

For some of you reading today, healing might take an entire lifetime. Yet again, no mind can imagine how

God chooses to heal. It is all counted as progress. I have thought deeply about the after-cancer experience. "What does life look like now? Is this healing?" If you saw me at a grocery store or running errands, my appearance would be nothing memorable or special. Our family has adjusted to normalcy as much as possible. Alex and I both work, and Sal has school. We face all life's daily decisions and little frustrations; what to make for dinner every night, cleaning up the messy kitchen, doing

For some of you reading today, healing might take an entire lifetime.

laundry over and over, and getting homework done at a reasonable hour. Yet still, our lives can never go back to what it was before cancer. I don't know what more will come in the future, but I know fully that God hears our requests and listens. God is still doing miracles today, *"What no eye has seen, what now ear has heard, and what no human mind has conceived -the things God has prepared for those who love him..." 1 Corinthians 2: 9 NIV*

It really is a mystery why God used figs to heal King Hezekiah or had to spit on the blind man's eyes twice. Or, why couldn't God have just healed Alex and Sal with a word? We know through scripture that God can heal by the power of His word. For those reading today, my prayer for you is God is at work, and He will heal your child. And please remember, don't lose hope because sometimes healing…*takes more than one dose.*

We count it all as progress. We move forward in joy, holding onto God's promise. *"What no eye has seen, what no ear has heard, and what no human mind has conceived -the things God has prepared for those who love him…"* 1 *Corinthians 2: 9 NIV*

The Scars that Remain

Suddenly Jesus was standing there among them!

"Peace be with you," he said. As he spoke, he showed them the wounds in his hands and his side.

They were filled with joy when they saw the Lord.

John 20: NLT

I want to pause and think about the scars. Jesus shows his disciplines his scars, and they are filled with joy. In the same way, I see the scar on Sal's body where his port was, and I am filled with joy. I recognize the journey he went through, and it represents victory. His port was the primary way of getting chemo into the body directly into the bloodstream. The port was under the skin, except there were three tiny dots you could see and feel, which stuck out slightly. There are a variety of places to put a port. Sal's port was on his upper right torso above his chest. One of the final steps toward VICTORY is when the port finally comes out through surgery. This port has been his chemo lifeline for over three years.

All that will remain is a scar in the shape of an uneven line on the body. It was a successful surgery. I cherish the thought that never again will chemo go through that port. Praise the Lord. A glimpse of victory! We celebrate this moment with joy. The hospital staff was all smiles, and the doctor even said, "These are my favorite days when we get to take out the port." I can't help to think – Are there other scars unseen that will remain? I am sure there will be, and time will tell. I know we can all point to marks on our own bodies where we endured something that left a scar. Reflect on a blemish or wound on your body. What does it remind you of? Does it represent bravery, a memory, or even hurt and pain? I see Sal's warrior scar as a gentle reminder of his battle, the sacrifice, and ultimately the healing from cancer.

I have been encouraged by a song recently written by Casting Crowns, "*Scars in Heaven.*" In the lyrics, they share, "*...the only scars in heaven won't belong to me and you. ...The only scars in heaven are the hands that hold you now.*" Wow!! I had not thought from that perspective before. Will Sal have his scar in heaven? Scripture shares with us Jesus showing himself to his disciples after the resurrection and points to the scars where the nails were. A gentle reminder of the battle against evil, God's ultimate sacrifice, and healing for all humanity that comes through His unending grace and forgiveness.

Thank you, Lord, for your scars–through them, we are victorious.

You Have Been Here Long Enough

"The Lord our God said to us at Horeb, 'You have stayed long enough at this mountain'"

Deuteronomy 1:6 NIV

In Chapter 1 of this book, we started on a mountain with Moses. I heard the nurse's words ringing in my ear, "You can't wait. You must go now! Get moving, go!' What mountain are you on right now? God is reminding us that we have stayed long enough. We find ourselves on another mountain after cancer. *"The Lord, our God said to us at Horeb, 'You have stayed long enough at this mountain.'" Deuteronomy 1:6 NIV*

We have entered a new transition, and it's time for a new mountain and to embrace the after-cancer experience. Maybe you are here too and not sure where to go? Maybe it is too soon, but that's ok. There will be a time to pivot and give yourself permission to move forward but never forget what you have experienced. I am changed, you are changed, and we can never go back to the way it was before. We hold onto the flicker of *hope* that may have now grown into a blazing flame. Cancer never wins. Whether that be earthly healing or heavenly healing, it's all healing. We have the Victory!

I remember when my Dad was in the ICU before he died and went to heaven. My mom and I were walking down the somber hallway with the white walls. The ICU was quiet. In front of us was a cleaning lady with dark hair pulled back in a bun. She was pushing two large trash bins. I noticed her eyes; for some reason, she just stopped in front of us and looked intently into us. She had long fingers, and with her pointer finger, she slowly pointed upward to heaven with a peaceful motion and a loving and calm smile. She said, "Heaven is our home; we are only renting here." It brought tremendous comfort and wisdom. She's right! My dad is home, and I find peace knowing he is in heaven. We are only renting here. If life is not feeling like it should, or maybe there is a feeling like, now what? We made it through the trial but now what? Was there purpose in this pain? Or maybe, you are a grieved parent and feeling lost in this world without your light.

> **This was never meant to be our home. We are only renting here, and we have a heavenly home waiting for us.**

The anger, grief, and sorrow are too heavy to carry. It's not the ending you expected. This was never meant to be our home. We are only renting here, and we have a heavenly home waiting for us. "*The Lord our God said to us, 'You have stayed long enough at this mountain.'*" *Deuteronomy 1:6 NIV* It is time to pivot and run your race. You are not alone. Go with God and keep the faith. We will dare to *hope* with you. Victory is ahead!

Conclusion

Victory is Ahead! What does it look like for you? What does it feel like for you? Here are my concluding thoughts. I had you in mind when I wrote this book. This is my experience to share with you so that you may know you are not alone. To share the flicker of hope towards healing for others and healing for myself. It takes courage to have hope in the most devastating news. Cancer will never win in the end.

Looking around at where I am now, I can confidently dare to hope. Let me be the one for you who was like the cleaning lady for us at the hospital. I want you to know I am pointing up! My finger is pointing to the sky, and I am cheering for you and your child. Let me be a reminder, heaven is our home! You can lift your head;

God's love abounds. There is hope. Victory is coming. I leave you with how this book started and a constant reminder of God's promise.

"The Lord himself goes before you and will be with you; he will never leave you nor forsake you. Do not be afraid; do not be discouraged."

Deuteronomy 31:8 NIV

For me, "Victory is Ahead" means not being gripped by fear or discouraged. My worry list is longer now than before cancer was part of our daily vernacular. But even if another cancer comes, even in death or relapses, I will not be afraid; the Lord is with me He is with you too. Yahweh reminds us, "*I am* always with you."

For me, "Victory is Ahead" means we will keep advocating for more research and better therapies so no parent has to hear the news, "Your child has cancer." We will keep being a voice for those who can't speak and a voice for all who share in our grief.

For me, "Victory is Ahead" means knowing God goes before us and is with us. There is nothing we can't do through Christ who strengthens us. The world can do its very worst. However, God will never forsake me, you, or your child. Our pain is never hidden.

For me, in a very tangible way, "Victory is Ahead" means swimming. Such an ordinary thing. What everyday things are on your victory list? What normal things were once constrained, and now you don't have to be as cautious? For us, swimming was one of many things Sal could not do during his treatments. For over three years, Sal just wanted to swim. He asked, "Mom and Dad, when I am done with chemo can we go somewhere and swim?" Absolutely my brave warrior! Swimming became a symbol of "victory" because it meant we could be finally free! Who would have thought swimming would be so treasured? So uncomplicated and straightforward, yet so freeing.

We planned a trip as a family to Great Wolf Lodge shortly after Sal was finished with all his chemo treatments. We dove into the water carefree and unafraid. So refreshing! It reminds me of baptism and God taking ordinary things, such as water, and doing something extraordinary. We are washed by the waters. An incredible gift from God.

God lovingly uses our ordinary lives, unique strengths, and incredible experiences and makes them extraordinary for His glory.

Victory Is Ahead

We have a God of peace (during uncertainty)

We have a God of joy (during sorrow)

We have a God of miracles (during pain)

Through Christ, you are Victorious,

Lisa

Appendix

Resources for Childhood Cancer Families

Disclaimer: No funds have been received from any of these organizations, and I do not have personal experience with all of them. But these are an accumulated list of resources from multiple sources.

Alex's Lemonade Stand Foundation: sibling program and educational material

American Childhood Cancer Organization

Comfycozy's for Chemo: Sends port shirts; usually tie-dye, and they have shirts and tunics.

Connor's Cuddles: Sends blankets to children in treatment for cancer

Costumes For Courage provides costumes to children receiving chemotherapy treatment

CURE Bears for Hope and Love: Sends Build A Bear Workshop bears and My Life Survivor dolls to children 0-12 years of age in treatment for cancer (limited to the United States)

Desi Strong Foundation: Sends dolls with a port to children in treatment for cancer

Evans Avengers: Creates awareness of the under-funding of Childhood Cancer Research, raises money for current research in all types of childhood cancers, and creates mentorships for the families during and after treatment

HopeKids: Provides ongoing events, activities, and a powerful, unique support community for families who have a child with cancer or some other life-threatening medical condition.

Hug Your People: Sends wagons to children in treatment for cancer to ease hospital visits.

Jars of Hope Inspired by Caroline: Sends a jar of toys and handmade pillowcase to kids across the United

States who are battling any medical issue and are ages 3-12 years

JZips: Sends port shirts, usually purchased at Target or Carters, that a cancer teen and his family can add two zippers on for easy access

Lighthouse Family Retreat: Offers restorative retreats and helpful resources

Love Your Melon: Provides a hat for girls or boys in treatment

Luke's FastBreaks: Provides port/medical shirts. They have snaps along both sides bottom of the shirt to the side of the sleeve.

Make-A-Wish: Helps fulfill the wishes of children with a critical illness between the ages of 2½ and 18 years old.

Our Amazing Fighters: Sends custom blankets and care packages to children in treatment for cancer.

Roc Solid Foundation: Donates book bags full of supplies for inpatient families, donate backyard play sets to kids, and ships them to their family (these need to be built by families and friends).

The Gold Hope Project: Offers photos of the child with cancer and their family for free.

Wipe Out Kids Cancer: Giving hope and support. Warrior Program, Buddy Bag program (North Texas), and Research Program.

About the Author

Elisa Marchetti (Lisa) will encourage you through her unique writing style of storytelling and personification. She interweaves scripture and God's promises throughout each chapter and will inspire you through her authentic and vulnerable experiences. Lisa is a gifted speaker and organizational effectiveness human resources leader who passionately supports multiple non-profit Childhood Cancer organizations. She will keep advocating for research and better therapies, so no parent has to hear the words, "Your child has cancer." Lisa lives with her husband and son in the Dallas, Texas, area.

Visit Lisa at: victoryisahead.com